MW00560002

ORTHOPEDICS

made
ridiculously
simple

Patrice Tétreault, MD, MSc, FRCSC

Assistant Professor
Orthopedic Surgery
CHUM—Pavillon Notre-Dame
University of Montreal

Hugue Ouellette, MD, FRCPC

Director of Education
Musculoskeletal Radiology
Massachusetts General Hospital
Harvard Medical School

MedMaster, Inc., Miami Florida

Copyright © 2014, 2013, 2010, 2009 by MedMaster, Inc.

All rights reserved. This book is protected by copyright. No part of it may be reproduced, stored in a retrieval system, or transmitted in any form or by any means, electronic, mechanical, photocopying, recording or otherwise, without written permission from the copyright owner.

Second Printing, 2009. Third Printing, 2010. Fourth Printing, 2013. Fifth Printing, 2014.

ISBN10# 0-940780-86-0
ISBN13# 978-0-940780-86-6

Made in the United States of America

Published by MedMaster, Inc.
P.O. Box 640028
Miami FL 33164

Cover illustration by Richard March

To my wife Jenny and children: Satia, Téodor and Mattéas.
Patrice Tétreault, M.D.

To my daughters Emanuelle and Gabrielle.
Hugue Ouellette, M.D.

ACKNOWLEDGMENTS

Geneviève Adam, medical student

William S. Allen, medical resident

Louis-Philippe Amiot, orthopedic surgeon

Marie-Andrée Cantin, pediatric orthopedic surgeon

Michèle Ciampini, administrative assistant, Orthopedic service

Sabrina Ciampini, student

Nicola Hagemeister, Ph.D.

Nicolas G. Hamelin, medical student

Marc Isler, Orthopedics Program Director, University of Montreal

Seth Jerabek, orthopedics resident

Alain Jodoin, Orthopedics Division Chief, University of Montreal

Alice Le, medical student

Jordan Leroux-Stewart, medical student

Annie Levasseur, biomechanics master student

Jae Oh, research assistant

Demetrios Rizis, medical student

Martin Torriani, musculoskeletal radiologist

CONTENTS

CHAPTER 3. LOWER LIMB 36

CONTENTS

ATLAS OF ORTHOPEDICS (http://www.medmaster.net)

PREFACE

This book was written with the intention of pursuing Dr. Stephen Goldberg's vision to make learning ridiculously simple. The reader will quickly acquire basic knowledge for the diagnosis and management of common orthopedic conditions encountered in the emergency room and the general practitioner's office. Although this book is intended for medical students and interns, it is also useful for nurses, nurse practitioners and medical assistants.

This small text is not meant to cover all of orthopedics in depth. It provides a broad overview of key areas that everyone should know about. For example, the first chapter addresses general concepts and principles in the diagnosis and management of common musculoskeletal injuries; it describes orthopedic emergencies and relevant clinical signs no one should miss. The subsequent chapters address the upper and lower limbs, the axial skeleton, systemic conditions affecting the musculoskeletal system, and common pediatric conditions. Each topic is covered with regards to the relevant anatomy, the clinical approach, and specific problems not to be overlooked.

This book offers the opportunity to consult an Atlas of Orthopedics that is available as a free download from www.medmaster.net. This will enable the reader to access many radiologic and orthopedic images and movies.

For the writing of this book, many hours were spent in the bookstores of Harvard Square in Boston. Young students rolling in with their suitcases brought back memories of medical school and the hard days of learning stuff as rapidly as possible. We also remember that humor is by far the best way to make learning enjoyable and memorable. We hope this book can provide a fun way to learn about orthopedics.

We would like to acknowledge the editing work done by Dr. Jenny C. Lin and the support of our institutions: Centre Hospitalier de l'Université de Montréal (CHUM), Division of Orthopedic Surgery, University of Montreal, and the Massachusetts General Hospital, Department of Radiology.

Patrice Tétreault, M.D.
Hugue Ouellette, M.D.

CHAPTER 1.   MUSCULOSKELETAL BASICS

I. TERMINOLOGY

To better understand the clinical orthopedic conditions described in this book, familiarize yourself with the following terms:

A. Orientation in Space (Fig. 1-1)

Anatomical position: The human body with the palms of the hands and the dorsum of the feet facing forward.

Midline: Central vertical axis of the body.
Medial: Close to the midline.
Lateral: Away from the midline.
Proximal: Closer to the head.
Distal: Farther from the head.
Palmar (volar): Palm side of the hand.
Plantar: Underside of the foot.
Sectional cuts: Sectional planes of the body used mainly for description of imaging studies (**Fig. 1-2**).

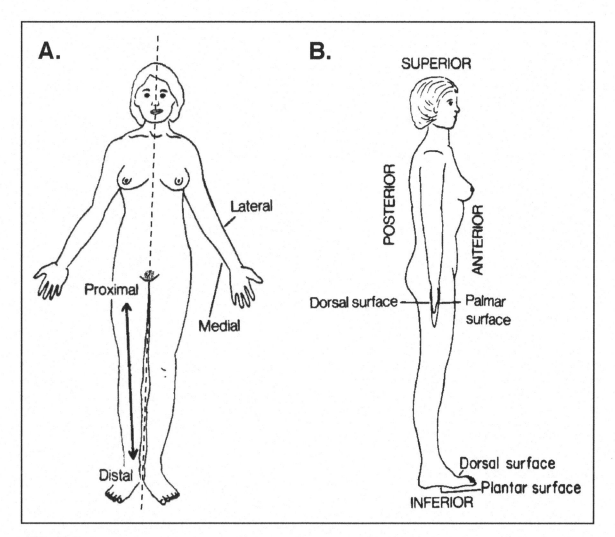

Fig. 1-1 Orientation in space. A: Anatomical position with midline (dashed line). **B:** Lateral view.

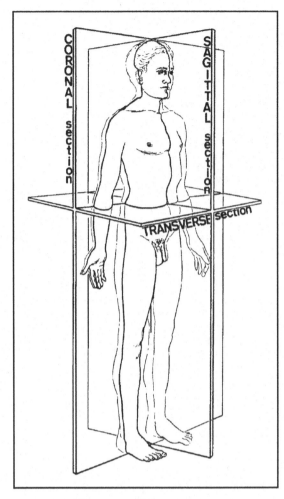

Fig. 1-2 Sectional cuts.

B. Movement in Space (Fig. 1-3)

ABduction: Movement of a limb away from midline.
ADduction: Movement of a limb close to midline.
Pronation: Forearm moving from anatomical position to palm facing posteriorly.
Supination: Forearm moving from palm facing posteriorly back into anatomical position (palm facing forward).
Flexion: Movement consisting of bending a joint.
Extension: Movement consisting of straightening a joint.
Eversion of the ankle: Rotation of the ankle outward.
Inversion of the ankle: Rotation of the ankle inward.

C. General Orthopedic Terms

Consolidation: To describe a healed fracture.
Flexum: Lack or deficit of extension in the range of motion of an articulation.

ORIF: Open Reduction Internal Fixation (reduction done after opening the skin).
Reduction: Action to reposition a deformed limb into anatomical alignment.
Sprain: Tearing of a ligament.
Strain: Tearing of a musculo-tendinous unit (remember with "**t**" in strain and tendon).
Valgus: Deformation of limb away from the body midline (remember with "**l**" as in **l**ateral).
Varus: Deformation of a limb toward the body midline (remember with "**r**" as in **r**ound).

II. MUSCULOSKELETAL CONDITIONS

A. General Approach

1. *Primary assessment—"ABC"*

Whenever a clinician evaluates a patient involved in an accident or a patient lying unconscious, the reflex should be to perform a formal primary assessment of the ABC's of life support, which are:

AIRWAY

BREATHING

CIRCULATION

In other words, vital organs of the body will fail without clear airways, proper inflow and outflow of air to the lungs, and a palpable arterial pulse, which means a functioning heart pumping an adequate blood volume. Although beyond the scope of this book, we encourage all clinicians to review the Advanced Cardiac Life Support (ACLS) and Advanced Trauma Life Support (ATLS) manuals, which address the techniques to support a deficient Airway, Breathing, or Circulation.

2. *Secondary assessment—"Symptoms and Signs"*

History

To make a correct clinical diagnosis, start by carefully listening to the patient's complaint. The patient will verbalize the problem in common terms, describing what was perceived using all senses (to feel, to see, to hear, to smell, and to taste). In other words, the patient will describe **SYMPTOMS** (e.g., felt pain, saw a bruise, heard a clunk, smelled bad, tasted yucky!).

Although pain is often the main complaint that brings patients to consult a doctor, it is a subjective symptom often difficult to define, express, or measure. Pain is also not perceived equally from one individual to another. The description of the pain should be thoroughly and precisely documented. Key questions are: How did

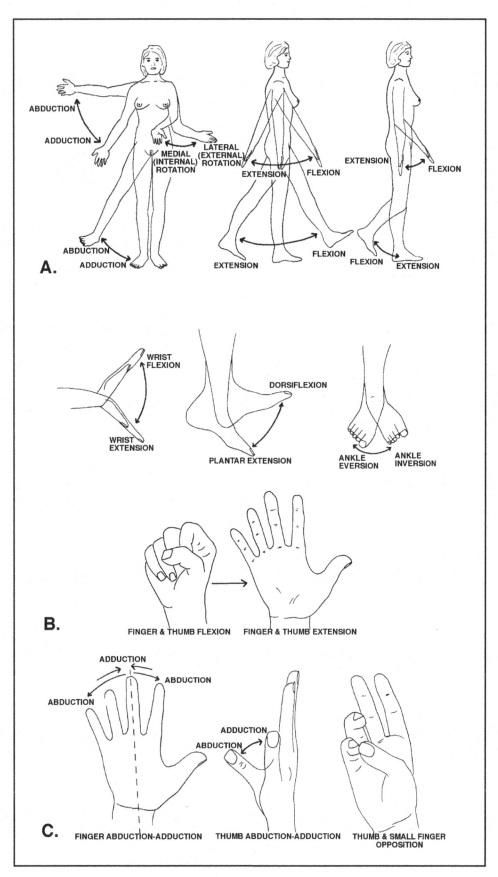

Fig. 1-3 Movement in space. A: Movement of the limbs. **B:** Movement of the hand and foot. **C:** Movement of the fingers.

the pain start? Where is the pain localized? What type of pain is experienced (burning, sharp . . .)? What makes it worse or better? Does the pain radiate somewhere? Does it hurt anywhere else?

The type of pain can also orient the clinician. A dull ache at the joint level suggests a local pathology, whereas a burning or tingling sensation suggests a nerve-related condition (neuropathy). Pain at rest relieved by movement indicates an inflammatory condition. Night pain is typical for inflammatory conditions. Pain upon effort relieved by rest suggests a mechanical pathology such as arthritis. Pain that is not increased by movement of the joint may originate from another area (referred pain).

The functional capacity of the patient can be determined by inquiring about the performance of activities of daily living (getting dressed, lifting objects, walking, sports . . .).

Physical Exam

Once the symptoms are well documented, look for evidences or **SIGNS** that a clinical condition is indeed present. Imagine yourself as a CSI agent (Clinical Signs Investigator) and examine the patient using the "**I** Personally **M**ake **S**ure and **C**heck" approach:

1. **I**nspection
2. **P**alpation
3. **M**obility (active and passive range of motion)
4. **S**pecialized maneuvers
5. **C**omplementary exams

For most orthopedic conditions, the physical exam will determine if the symptoms (pain mostly) are truly coming from a joint (articular), from around the joint (periarticular), or from a distant location (referred pain, such as a lumbar disk hernia causing foot pain).

Inspection

The inspection can start as soon as the patient enters the examination room. Take the opportunity to look at general posture and gait. When asking the patient to undress, examine the supposedly painful limb, since patients seeking insurance compensation may momentarily forget to feign their illness. It is also useful to look repetitively at the normal limb and injured limb to pick up subtle signs of asymmetry, such as swelling, muscle atrophy, and discoloration.

Palpation

The palpation gives the opportunity to feel for swelling, articular effusion, warmth, crepitus, and snapping.

Mobility

Assessment of the range of motion of a limb or spine will give a good idea of the loss of function. Start with active range of motion by asking the patient to move the desired body part to the maximal possible amplitude. Assess passive range of motion by moving the body part for the patient to reach maximal amplitude or level at which the pain is unbearable. The type of stiffness can be very informative for the clinician. With inflammatory pathologies (e.g., rheumatoid arthritis), stiffness is classically in the morning. It is usually severe and long lasting (>1 hour). With mechanical pathologies (e.g. osteoarthritis), morning stiffness is less severe and lasts a short time. It is worse during the day after a brief period of rest.

The loss of function that results from structural damage to a joint or limb can also vary significantly. With articular pathologies, the active and passive ranges of motion are usually limited. For most periarticular pathologies, the active range of motion is limited, but the passive range of motion is normal. For most referred pain pathologies, the examination of the joint is usually normal.

Specialized maneuvers

Specialized maneuvers are performed to rule out a suspected condition. Generally, the examiner stresses specific tendons or ligaments to evaluate the loss of function. We will discuss specialized maneuvers with the corresponding orthopedic condition. With articular pathologies, movements against resistance are pain free. For most periarticular pathologies, movement against resistance will reproduce the pain.

Complementary exams

The complementary exams consist of tests done with specialized tools to have a closer look at the body. They also help confirm clinical suspicion. The tests may include blood work (hemoglobin, white blood cell count), cultures of various fluids, radiographs, nuclear bone scan, CT scan, magnetic resonance imaging (MRI), and many others. For all orthopedic conditions described throughout this book, the most appropriate complementary exam to be ordered will be mentioned.

B. Radiology

Musculoskeletal injuries are often investigated with radiographs to rule out an underlying fracture. Radiographs of the joint above and below the level of a fracture should always be obtained to exclude intra-articular extension of the fracture.

Keep in mind the "X- ray rule of 2's":

–2 views: Antero-Posterior (AP) and lateral of the injured area
–2 joints: joint above and joint below the injured area

–2 times: before and after a reduction or manipulation
–2 sides: bilateral x-rays of the injured and uninjured
 limbs for comparison

Additional tests such CT, MRI, and bone scan are helpful in particular conditions and will be added to the list of required tests when necessary. CT scans are particularly good for assessment of bones. MR imaging is most helpful for soft tissue injury assessment. Bone scan is important for assessment of increased bone turnover.

When in doubt about the presence of a fracture, consult textbooks or a radiologist to confirm your findings. This is the best method to build expertise with radiographs.

C. Fractures and Dislocations

The orthopedic surgeon will listen carefully when a fracture is described over the phone since he or she will try to distinguish a benign condition that can wait until the next clinic, from a true emergency. Fractures can be described as follows:

Fracture types (Fig. 1-4)

Simple fracture: The fracture results in 2 bony fragments.
Spiral fracture: The fracture line is oblique and looks like the sign of a barber shop.

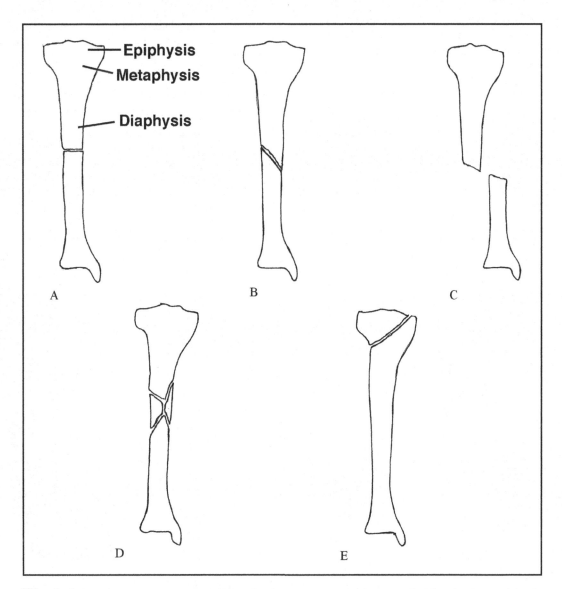

Fig. 1-4 Basic fracture types. A: Non-displaced transverse fracture. **B:** Non-displaced oblique fracture. **C:** Displaced oblique fracture. **D:** Comminuted fracture. **E:** Intra-articular fracture.

Transverse fracture: The fracture line is perpendicular to the long axis of the bone.

Non-displaced fracture: The bony fragments are in contact with each other and normally aligned.

Displaced fracture: The bony fragments are misaligned.

Comminuted fracture: The fracture results in 3 or more bony fragments.

Extra-articular fracture: The fracture line does not cross the articular surface of a joint.

Intra-articular fracture: The fracture line crosses the articular surface of a joint.

Dislocation: Loss of the normal alignment of a joint such that the articular surfaces are not in contact with one another.

To add more precision to the description, most bones with an elongated shape can be subdivided in 3 sections: *Epiphysis* (tip), *Metaphysis* (funnel shaped area), *Diaphysis* (shaft).

Fracture Healing

The healing of a fracture requires that the bony fragments be in contact or in very close proximity, and involves the formation of a bridging structure called a *callus*. Intuitively, if a large gap is present between the fragments due to soft tissue interposition, the fracture has little chance of forming any callus. The callus is fragile and must be protected with immobilization of the limb. If there is motion at the fracture site, the bony bridges will break and the fracture may take longer to heal (delayed union) or may not heal at all (non-union). Fracture consolidation of large bones usually takes 6 to 8 weeks in the adult.

In summary, requirements for proper fracture healing are:

1. Close proximity of fracture fragments
2. Immobilization
3. Time

Fracture Management

A traumatized limb must be immobilized as soon as possible to decrease pain and to avoid aggravation of soft tissue injuries. All deformed limbs, which may have a fracture, must be correctly aligned by gently pulling on the limb (axial traction). Use a plaster (or synthetic resin) slab to splint the limb before sending for x-rays (**Fig. 1-5**).

Conservative approach. Non-displaced fractures are generally treated with immobilization in a cast.

Cast technique. The fractured limb is wrapped gently with soft roll. Plaster rolls are submerged in water to activate the chemical process for hardening. Excess water is removed by squeezing the roll, which is then snugly unrolled over the fractured limb. As a general principle,

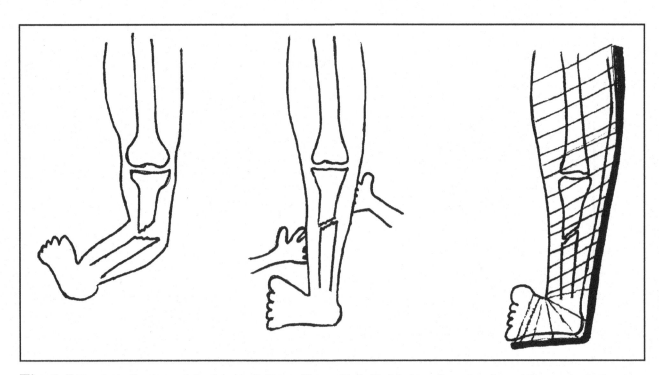

Fig. 1-5 Basic splinting of the leg. A: Deformed lower limb. **B:** Limb realignment by gentle manipulation. **C:** Limb splinting.

make sure to span the fracture site with plaster including the joint above and the joint below the fracture to provide enough stability for fracture healing. Specific details for cast technique for the different bone fractures will be mentioned in the corresponding section in the book. Help provided by an orderly to support the injured limb may be required. The application of a cast is an art by itself and proper skills can be taught by a plaster technician or an orthopedic surgeon in hospitals or seminars.

Non-displaced intra-articular fractures can also be treated in this manner. Slightly displaced extra-articular fractures are realigned with gentle manipulation (reduction) and are immobilized with a cast. Close follow-up with weekly radiographs will ensure that they stay in an acceptable position.

Surgical approach. Surgery is considered for cases where the fracture fragments have no chance of forming bony bridging (large gap) or could heal in a poor position (mal-union). In other words, surgery is reserved for irreducible and unstable fractures. The fracture fragments are realigned surgically (*open reduction*) and immobilized with plates, screws, and/or wires (*internal fixation*). This process is referred to as *ORIF* (*Open Reduction Internal Fixation*). Intra-articular fractures with a step-off deformity of the articular surface of more than 2mm require anatomic reduction with ORIF to prevent late complications such as post-traumatic arthritis caused by the incongruent articular surfaces.

Dislocations

A dislocation of a joint is an emergency and must be reduced as soon as possible. Reduction maneuvers are attempted in the emergency room, usually with mild sedation. If the reduction is unsuccessful, the patient must be brought to the operating room for a reduction under general anesthesia with the possibility of an open reduction.

III. EMERGENCIES

There are three common orthopedic emergencies. Don't be "CONned" by the subtle signs of these emergencies (nicknamed "**CON**" lesions), which are: **C**ompartment syndrome, **O**pen fractures, **N**eurological/vascular injuries. If suspected, "CON" also means:

"**C**all **O**rtho **N**ow!!!"

A. Compartment Syndrome

Muscle groups are enclosed and separated from each other by a thick, non-elastic fascia. Any circumstance that increases the pressure in the compartment can eventually lead to inadequate perfusion of tissues within that compartment (ischemia). This is called a *compartment syndrome.* If this situation is not corrected, there is soft tissue death (necrosis), which may lead to functional disabilities or loss of the limb. There are two main causes of this increase in compartment pressure: 1) an increase in the contents of the compartment (i.e., bleeding and swelling of the muscle) or 2) decreased volume of the compartment (cast or bandage too tight). The sensitivity of the soft tissues to ischemia varies, with nerves dying first, followed by muscles. The threshold for a compartment syndrome may vary from one patient to another (i.e., hypotensive patients are more at risk due to poor perfusion pressure).

Clinical Findings

The *5 P's:*

1. **Pain:** Pain out of proportion to the injury despite adequate analgesia is the most reliable indicator of compartment syndrome (most sensitive sign). The pain, due to muscle ischemia, is particularly exquisite with movement of the affected muscle compartment.
2. **Paresthesia:** Numbness is the first sign of peripheral nerve ischemia.
3. **Palpation:** The compartment becomes hard and tense in comparison with the opposite side.
4. **Paralysis:** The patient cannot move the muscles in that compartment.
5. **Pallor and/or Pulselessness:** This sign is the least reliable for diagnosis (least sensitive sign), since the pressure required to occlude the arterial pulse is much higher than that needed to affect the viability of the soft tissues.

Do not wait until the pulse is gone to suspect and treat a compartment syndrome!

Intra-compartmental pressure measurement can be made with a specialized instrument for definitive diagnosis. Generally, a compartment pressure over 30 mmHg is diagnostic. One should also remember that there must always be greater than 15 mmHg difference between the patient's diastolic pressure and the compartment pressure to allow perfusion of that compartment.

Treatment

Clinical SUSPICION is the key. Consult a surgeon without delay to confirm the diagnosis. With the agreement of the surgeon, open all casts and bandages until the skin is visible. If the symptoms persist, the surgeon must proceed to open the fascia (fasciotomy) to decrease the pressure within the compartment.

A possible complication of a compartment syndrome is fibrous scarring of the tissues, causing loss of function and contracture deformity of the involved muscle group. This is called *Volkmann's contracture,* and can be a devastating outcome of compartment syndrome.

B. Open Fractures

An open fracture implies that the skin is perforated and that bone was brought into contact with bacteria in the environment through a visible wound. This increases the likelihood of a bone infection (osteomyelitis), which is very hard to cure. The bigger the wound is, the higher the risk of infection. The notion of time is also extremely important. The longer a wound is exposed to the environment, the greater the risk of infection. Therefore, one must find out the precise time the accident actually happened.

In the Emergency Room (ER)

The treatment of an open fracture is urgent. It must begin immediately with superficial cleaning of the wound and surrounding skin with sterile water and coverage with a sterile dressing.

An open fracture requires immediate antibiotic coverage. The choice of antibiotics depends on wound size and duration of exposure (**Fig. 1-6**).

Classification of Open Fractures (Gustillo and Anderson)

Type I: Wound size of less than 1 cm resulting from protrusion of a bone spike through the skin.

Type II: Wound size between 1 to 10 cm resulting from high energy trauma.

Type III a: Wound size over 10 cm without periosteal stripping or loss of soft tissue coverage.

b: Wound size over 10 cm with loss of soft tissue coverage requiring skin grafting.

c: Wound size over 10 cm with loss of blood perfusion to the affected limb.

Even with a very small wound, the patient must be protected against tetanus (Td). Tetanus comes from a toxin produced by the bacterium *Clostridium tetani*. It can cause severe neurological symptoms such as muscular spasms and ultimately DEATH! For proper tetanus coverage, one must consider the patient's prior vaccination status (**Fig. 1-7**).

In the Operating Room (OR)

The surgeon will clean the wound and bone, and remove all dead tissues. The fracture will be reduced and immobilized. The wound may be left open and debrided as often as necessary in subsequent operations. A consultation with a plastic surgeon may be necessary when a large wound requires a skin graft or muscle flap for closure.

C. Neurological/Vascular Injury

All fractures or dislocations present a risk for neurological and vascular injury.

Clinical Findings

Symptoms and signs of a neurological injury include altered or absent sensation in the territory of an injured nerve and loss of muscular contraction. Signs of a vascular injury include asymmetry in limb color, delayed capillary refill, and a weak or absent pulse. Capillary refill means that when you press on the soft tissues of the distal fingers or toes, it takes a second or two before the whitened skin returns to pink. If the capillary refill takes more then three second, it is said to be delayed.

Treatment

In the presence of a suspected injury to a peripheral nerve, **consult a plastic surgeon without delay.** The surgeon will order electromyography (EMG) studies and follow the patient for a possible spontaneous recovery. The plastic surgeon may alternatively opt for surgical repair.

There are three types of nerve injuries, which are in order of increasing severity:

1. *Neurapraxia* (sleepy nerve): The nerve conduction is interrupted due to localized trauma to the nerve and surrounding tissues. The axons and myelin sheath of the nerve are still intact. Therefore, the recovery from the loss of function of a nerve can be quick (minutes) or slow (months) depending on the trauma.

2. *Axonotmesis:* The axons of the nerve are cut, but the myelin sheet is intact. The axons beyond the location of the nerve injury degenerate after the trauma, but the intact myelin sheath allows for regeneration of the axons up to the muscle. The functional recovery is almost complete. A nerve can grow back through the myelin sheath 1 millimeter per day. Knowing the length of the nerve from the injury site up to the muscle, one can calculate the time for recovery. No surgery is required, just observation.

3. *Neurotmesis:* The axons and the myelin sheath were cut at the time of injury. There is usually a wound close to the site of nerve injury. The only possible treatment is surgical reattachment of the nerve ends. The recovery is possible but less predictable than neurapraxia and axonotmesis due to the scar tissue interfering with nerve regeneration.

In the presence of a suspected vascular injury, simple realignment or traction on the limb may restore the perfusion. If the limb remains pale or pulseless, consult a vascular surgeon without delay. The surgeon will order an angiogram to locate the injury and then attempt a repair.

In summary, with a systematic approach, orthopedic conditions encountered at the office or emergency room can be diagnosed and treated with the appropriate level of urgency, and referred to a specialist when needed.

Open fracture	In the ER	On the ward*
Type I/ II	Ancef 2 g IV stat	Ancef 1 g IV q8h for 3 days
Type III †	Ancef 2 g IV and Gentamycin 2 mg/kg IV stat	Ancef 2 g IV and Gentamycin 1-2 mg/kg IV q8h for 3 days
Any type with

Farm injury or Vascular injury | Ancef 2 g IV and Gentamycin 2 mg/kg IV and Penicillin 10 million units stat | Ancef 2 g IV and Gentamycin 1-2 mg/kg IV q8h for 3 days and Penicillin 10 million units/day for 3 days |

*Repeat antibiotic therapy for 3 days after each additional surgical intervention.
† Included type I/II if time of injury more than 6 hours.

Fig. 1-6 Guidelines for antibiotic prophylaxis

History of tetanus immunization (doses)	Clean minor wounds		Other wounds	
	Give Td	Give TIG*	Give Td	Give TIG*
Unknown or less than 3 doses	Yes	No	Yes	Yes
3 doses or more	No (Yes if > 10 years since last dose)	No	No (Yes if > 5 years since last dose)	No

* TIG (tetanus immune globulin) given with toxoid at separate sites 250 units IM

Fig. 1-7 Guidelines for tetanus prophylaxis

CHAPTER 2. UPPER LIMB

I. SHOULDER

The shoulder joint is much like the game of golf. A ball (humeral head) stable on the tee (scapula) is the first step to decrease your handicap.

A. Anatomy

The glenohumeral joint is analogous to a golf ball resting on a golf tee as seen from an axillary view (**Fig. 2-1**). The shoulder joint is in fact composed of 3 synovial joints: the *sternoclavicular, acromioclavicular* and *glenohumeral* joints (**Fig. 2-2**). The glenohumeral ligaments are attached to the *labrum,* which is a cartilaginous donut that surrounds the glenoid rim. They form the shoulder joint capsule, which provides stability to the glenohumeral joint (**Fig. 2-3**). Half of the arm elevation is provided by motion at the glenohumeral joint. Full arm elevation requires motion at the scapulothoracic level with rotation of the scapula over the ribs (**Fig. 2-4**).

Pretend you are holding a golf ball between your fingers. Your fingers are analogous to the rotator cuff muscles attached to the humeral head. The index finger represents the long head of the biceps. Other fingers represent the rotator cuff muscles. As the golf ball "SITS" between your fingers, use the "SITS" acronym to remember the rotator cuff muscles (**Fig. 2-5**). Rotating the ball between your fingers (as if reading the name on the ball) is analogous to the function of the rotator cuff on

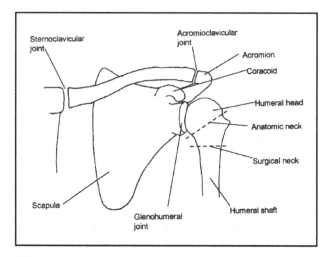

Fig. 2-2 Shoulder anatomy.

the humeral head (**Fig. 2-6**). The muscle that shapes the contour of the shoulder is the deltoid muscle (**Fig. 2-7**).

B. Approach

Sudden pain usually suggests rotator cuff tendinitis or tendon tear. The pain classically presents at night. Localized pain to the acromioclavicular (AC) joint represents AC pathology, which is most likely arthritis. Pain to the level of the insertion of the deltoid muscle over the lateral aspect of the mid-humerus is classically

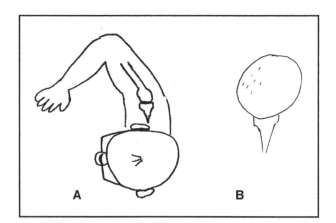

Fig. 2-1 Axillary view of the shoulder. A: Glenohumeral joint. **B:** Golf ball on a tee.

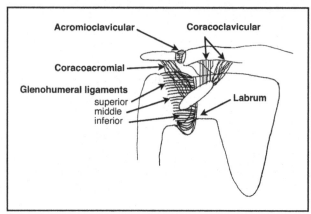

Fig. 2-3 Shoulder ligaments.

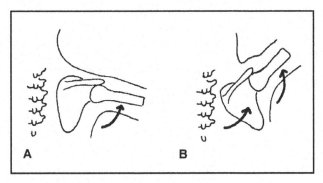

Fig. 2-4 A: Posterior view of mid-elevation with motion mainly at the glenohumeral joint. **B:** Full arm elevation with motion at both the glenohumeral joint and scapulothoracic levels.

a referred pain due to rotator cuff pathology. A constant intense pain (night and day), with limitation in the range of motion, mostly likely involves inflammation of the capsule (*capsulitis*), the synovial membrane (*synovitis*) or the articular surface (*glenohumeral arthritis*). The systemic symptom of fever makes septic arthritis more likely, whereas extra-articular manifestations, such as conjunctivitis, skin nodules, or psoriasis, can be signs of an inflammatory condition.

The physical examination is summarized below:

1. Inspection: –skin lesion
   –swelling
   –muscular atrophy

2. Range of motion:
   i) Active: –hand behind the head (to test abduction / external rotation)
   –hand behind the back (to test internal rotation)
   –circumduction (to test which motion cause pain)

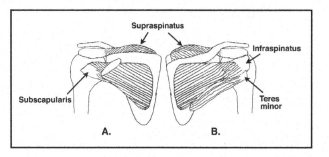

Fig. 2-6 Shoulder rotator cuff muscles. A: Anterior view. **B:** Posterior view.

   ii) Passive: –abduction alone
   –abduction with internal/external rotation
   –external rotation with elbow next to thorax

3. Palpation: –sternoclavicular joint
   –acromioclavicular joint
   –glenohumeral joint
   –periarticular (biceps tendon, rotator cuff, neck)

4. Specific maneuvers: –resist abduction (test supraspinatus)
   –resist external rotation (test infraspinatus/teres minor)
   –resist internal rotation (test subscapularis)
   –impingement maneuvers (cf. Impingement syndrome)
   –upper extremities reflexes

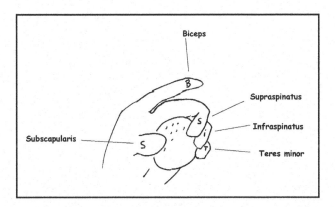

Fig. 2-5 Golf ball "SITS" between your fingers.

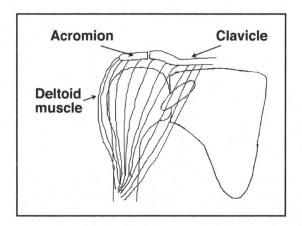

Fig. 2-7 Deltoid muscle.

C. Specific Problems

1. Impingement syndrome and rotator cuff tear

Imagine a golf club close to your fingers while you are holding a golf ball. The club is analogous to the acromion close to the rotator cuff (**Fig. 2-8**). Impingement syndrome relates to repetitive squeezing of the rotator cuff tendons between the acromion and the humeral head. This is analogous to repetitively hitting your fingers with the golf club. The result is chronic inflammation of the rotator cuff (bruised fingers), also referred to as *cuff tendinitis*. Impingement may eventually lead to a rotator cuff tear (**Fig. 2-9**).

A rotator cuff tear can involve one or more tendons. It can also occur after a fall or sudden strenuous effort to raise the arm; however, the majority of rotator cuff tears are degenerative.

Clinical Findings

Impingement pain radiates over the lateral side of the shoulder. Night pain is classic. Most patients are unable to perform repetitive motion with the arm overhead. Muscle atrophy around the scapula suggests a chronic rotator cuff tear. Weakness of arm elevation is present. Several clinical tests are used for diagnosis of impingement by trying to reproduce the patient's symptoms using provocative measures (**Fig. 2-10**).

Impingement maneuvers

- *Neer maneuver:* At maximal passive forward flexion of the arm, the examiner applies a light pressure to further flex the arm to press the rotator cuff against the acromion.
- *Hawkins maneuver:* 90 degrees of forward flexion of the arm with the elbow flexed at 90 degrees, the

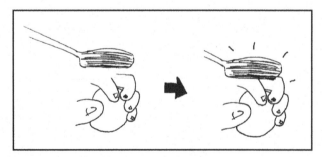

Fig. 2-8 Impingement syndrome. A golf club and fingers holding the ball are analogous to the acromion and the rotator cuff, respectively. A golf club hitting the fingers is analogous to impingement of the rotator cuff under the acromion.

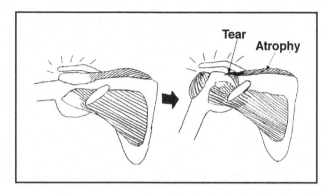

Fig. 2-9 Rotator cuff impingement. Rotator cuff impingement causes inflammation of the tendons (tendinitis). Eventually, the rotator cuff tears, causing retraction of the tendon and atrophy of the muscle.

examiner twists the arm with internal rotation to further press the rotator cuff against the acromion.
- *Empty beer can test:* test strength of the supraspinatus muscle against resistance. The arm is held at 90 degrees forward flexion, 30 degrees adduction, and internal rotation (thumb down much like emptying a beer can), and resisting downward force of the examiner.

Shoulder pain may originate from the cervical nerve being pinched. You can determine the origin of the pain by injecting a local anesthetic under the acromion (lidocaine test). Impingement pain will resolve whereas cervical pain will persist.

A simple AP X-ray may reveal a decreased acromiohumeral space, suggestive of rotator cuff thinning or tear. MRI is extremely sensitive for the detection of rotator cuff tendinitis and tear. It can also help in the evaluation of muscle atrophy.

Treatment

Conservative approach. The first line of treatment is activity modification, mainly avoiding repetitive overhead arm motion. Pain is managed with analgesics (NSAIDs) and steroid infiltration can help by diminishing inflammation. Physical therapy is used to strengthen the unaffected muscles of the rotator cuff, and this may help the affected tendon to recuperate.

Surgical approach. If a conservative approach fails after a 6 to 12 month period, surgery is considered. It consists of smoothing the undersurface of the acromion (acromioplasty) to provide more room for the rotator cuff tendons. Repair of a rotator cuff tear is done by suturing the tendon back to the humeral head. Recovery can be as long as 4 to 6 months. Strengthening therapy can be started at the third month post-op.

CHAPTER 2.   UPPER LIMB

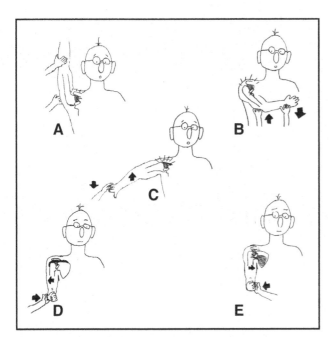

Fig. 2-10 Testing for rotator cuff tendinitis and tear. A: Neer sign maneuver to find impingement. **B:** Hawkins's maneuver to find impingement. **C:** Empty beer can test maneuver to find tendinitis or tear of the supraspinatus muscle. **D:** Testing external rotation strength of posterior cuff muscles (infraspinatus and teres minor muscles). **E:** Testing internal rotation strength of anterior cuff muscle (subscapularis muscle).

2. Adhesive capsulitis

Imagine that the golf ball is duct-taped to the tee. This is equivalent to the shoulder joint capsule (duct tape), which tightly joins the humeral head to the glenoid. Adhesive capsulitis is an inflammation of the shoulder capsule, such that the capsular volume shrinks and restricts motion (**Fig. 2-11**). It can occur spontaneously (idiopathic) or after events affecting the joint, such as fracture, infection, and traumatic rotator cuff tear. Diabetics are more prone to this condition.

Clinical Findings

The main symptoms are restricted range of motion in all planes and intense pain.

Therefore, all the provocative tests are inconclusive and not really useful.

X-rays are usually normal.

Treatment

Conservative approach. The pain usually fades after a few weeks, but the full range of motion takes a long

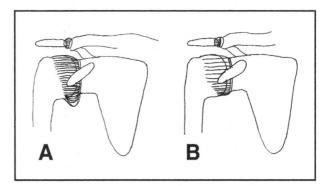

Fig. 2-11 Adhesive capsulitis. A: Normal joint capsule. **B:** Shrunken joint capsule.

time to regain. Spontaneous recovery can occur after 12 to 18 months. Physical therapy and intra-articular steroid injection can improve the symptoms and also accelerate the recovery.

Surgical approach. Surgery may be considered after 6 months of conservative treatment. This includes cutting the capsule (*capsulotomy*) by arthroscopy. The shoulder joint is then mobilized under anesthesia.

3. Proximal humeral fracture

A proximal humeral head fracture (broken golf ball) frequently occurs in the elderly. More violent traumas are required in young adults to create this fracture pattern.

Clinical Findings

Among the signs and symptoms of a proximal humeral fracture, axillary nerve injury must be ruled out. The latter presents with numbness on the lateral side of the shoulder and possibly weakness of the deltoid muscle.

An axillary view X-ray must be done to further determine the fracture configuration. There are several possible fracture configurations, according to the number of fragments (**Fig. 2-12**). A pre-operative CT scan can help the surgeon with surgical planning.

Treatment

Conservative approach. Slightly or non-displaced humeral head fractures are treated conservatively with sling immobilization for 3 weeks (**Fig. 2-12A**). Physiotherapy is started at 3 weeks for progressive mobilization.

Surgical approach. Fracture fragments displaced more than 1 cm or with severe angulation require ORIF (**Fig. 2-12B**). When the proximal humeral head is shattered, hemiarthroplasty is sometimes necessary (**Fig. 2-12C**).

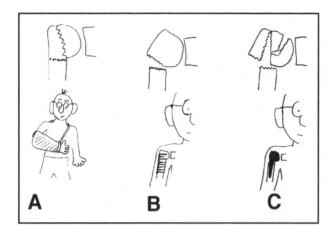

Fig. 2-12 Humeral head fracture. A: Non-displaced anatomical neck fracture (zigzag line) and surgical neck fracture (dotted line) treated with a sling. **B:** Displaced humeral head fracture treated with ORIF. **C:** Comminuted humeral head fracture treated with humeral head replacement prosthesis.

4. Clavicular fracture

Clavicular fractures are frequent in young adults. 80% are situated in the medial third of the clavicle.

Clinical Findings

A localized deformity may be mild to very pronounced. Rarely, there is numbness radiating to the hand due to brachial plexus compression.

Treatment

Conservative approach. The vast majority of patients can be treated with a figure-of-eight sling for comfort (**Fig. 2-13**).

Surgical approach. A wide displacement of the fracture fragments with no chance of union between the 2 bony ends needs ORIF (**Fig. 2-14**). Fractures of the distal third of the clavicle have a high incidence of non-union.

5. Acromioclavicular (AC) joint separation

AC joint separation implies that the clavicle is not aligned with the acromion. This injury is usually the result of a lateral impact on the shoulder, such as when a football player is tackled to the ground.

Clinical Findings

The pain and swelling is localized to the acromioclavicular (AC) joint. The distal end of the clavicle can

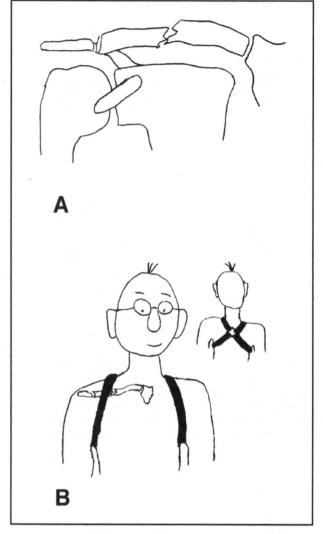

Fig. 2-13 Clavicle fracture. A: Slightly displaced clavicle fracture. **B:** Conservative treatment with figure-8 sling.

be elevated relative to the acromion and can be pressed down with the examiner's finger. This is referred to as the "piano key deformity."

X-ray views with the patient holding weights (5 lbs) in his or her hands can be done (stress radiographs). The weights accentuate AC joint malalignment. The right and left AC joint can be compared in more subtle cases. This injury is classified according to the extent of displacement (**Fig. 2-15**).

Grade I: There is pain and swelling with mobilization, but without instability on stress X-rays. This injury is a sprain of the ligaments of the acromioclavicular joint capsule.

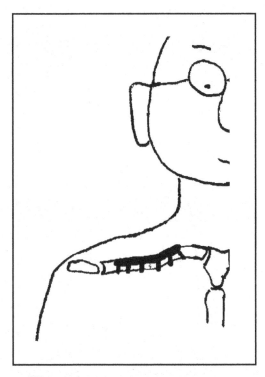

Fig. 2-14 Clavicle fracture ORIF.

Grade II: There is asymmetry of the injured AC joint on stress X-rays when compared to the AC joint of the normal shoulder. There is partial displacement of the distal clavicle relative to the acromion. This injury involves a tear in the ligaments of the AC joint capsule.

Grade III: A classic piano key deformity is present with complete AC joint dislocation. There is complete displacement of the distal clavicle relative to the acromion.

This injury implies tear of the joint capsule, and partial to complete rupture of the coracoclavicular ligaments.

Treatment

Conservative approach. For grade I, II and III, ice application and analgesics are recommended. The arm is kept in a sling for 2 to 3 weeks. The patient should then avoid heavy lifting for 2 months.

Surgical approach. Surgery is warranted when the dislocation is severe, when the patient is young, or when the patient is an athlete. It consists of repairing the AC joint capsule and the torn coracoclavicular ligaments. The repair can be further stabilized with a screw passing through the distal clavicle to the coracoid (**Fig. 2-16**).

For a chronic dislocation, excision of the distal clavicle is usually required to allow realignment of the remaining clavicle with the acromion. The original ligaments may be deficient such that reconstruction is done by detaching the acromial part of the coracoacromial ligament and transferring it to the distal end of the clavicle.

6. Glenohumeral joint dislocation

A glenohumeral joint dislocation is analogous to the golf ball falling off the tee (**Fig. 2-17**). Dislocations are common in young individuals involved in sports. For the joint to dislocate, structural damage must occur. The type of dislocation is described according to the position of the humeral head relative to the glenoid. Anterior dislocation is more common than posterior dislocation.

Clinical Findings

When the humeral head is dislocated anteriorly, internal rotation of the arm is impeded due to abutment of the humeral head on the anterior side of the glenoid.

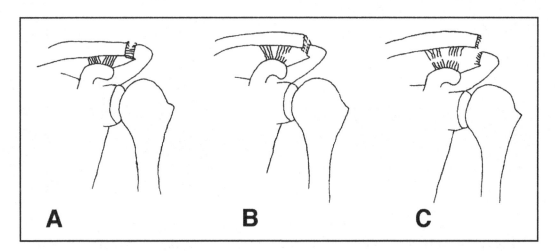

Fig. 2-15 Acromioclavicular dislocation types. A: Grade I. **B:** Grade II. **C:** Grade III.

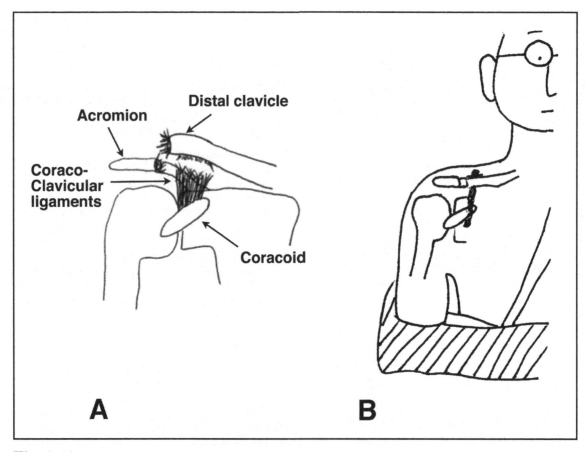

Fig. 2-16 Acromioclavicular dislocation. A: Grade III AC dislocation with over 100% displacement of the clavicle relative to the acromion. **B:** Stabilization of the AC joint with a screw passing through the distal clavicle and coracoid.

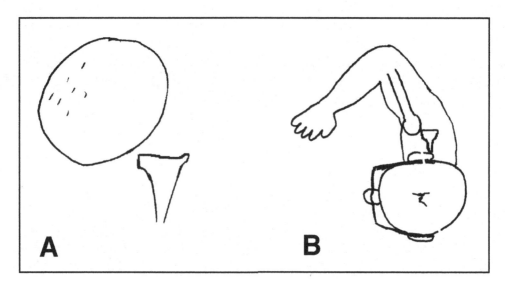

Fig. 2-17 Anterior shoulder dislocation. A: Golf ball off the tee. **B:** Humeral head off the glenoid.

With a posterior shoulder dislocation however, external rotation of the arm is restricted. A palpable bulge is present over the area where the humeral head is displaced, and a shallow depression is present on the opposite side. Numbness over the lateral side of the shoulder and possible paralysis of the deltoid muscle are due to axillary nerve stretching with anterior dislocation. A patient presenting with an unstable shoulder due to recurrent anterior dislocation will usually fear an impending dislocation when the arm is placed into abduction and full external rotation (*apprehension sign*).

AP and axillary X-ray views are required. The axillary view is the most reliable view to rule out an anterior or posterior dislocation. The impact of the glenoid rim on the dislocated humeral head can cause an indentation on the humeral head (*Hill-Sachs lesion*) (**Fig. 2-18A**). There may also be a glenoid rim fracture known as a *bony Bankart lesion* (**Fig. 2-18B**). Osseous injuries can be thoroughly assessed with CT scan. Usually the labrum and ligaments will tear off the glenoid edge (*cartilaginous Bankart lesion*). A cartilaginous Bankart lesion is best documented with MRI.

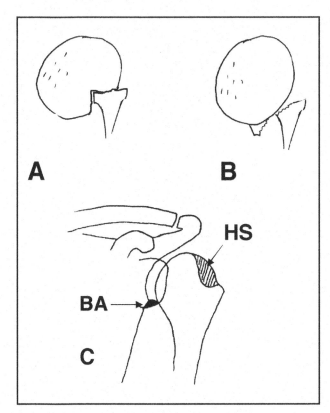

Fig. 2-18 Hill-Sachs and Bankart lesions. A: Broken golf ball analogous to Hill-Sachs lesion on the humeral head. **B:** Broken golf tee analogous to osseous Bankart lesion. **C:** Location of Bankart (BA) and Hill-Sachs (HS) lesions on scapula and humerus.

Treatment

Conservative approach. When a dislocation occurs for the first time, it usually requires an attempt at closed reduction in the emergency room (**Fig. 2-19**).

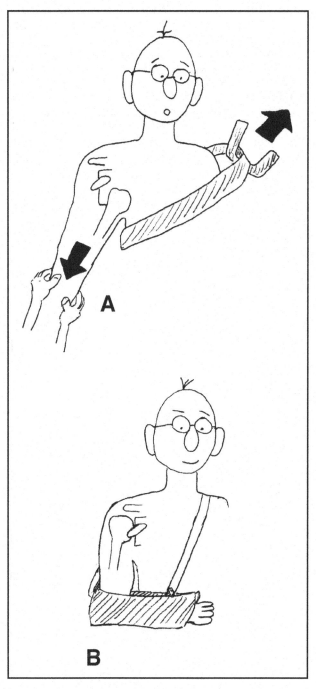

Fig. 2-19 Shoulder reduction. A: Reduction maneuver using a piece of fabric in the axilla. **B:** Reduced shoulder joint with arm in a sling.

Mild sedation is necessary and is usually given through an intravenous line. Shoulder reduction is performed by pulling on the arm (applying traction) to restore joint alignment. The pulling motion should be gentle and constant. A piece of fabric is wrapped around the torso to provide traction in the opposite direction. After a few minutes (up to 10 minutes) the muscles will relax and allow for reduction of the humeral head. General anesthesia is rarely needed.

Always document a successful reduction with an X-ray. After reduction, the shoulder is protected with a sling for 3 weeks to allow stretched or torn ligaments to heal. Physical therapy can then be initiated to strengthen the rotator cuff and other muscles around the scapula (shoulder girdle). The stability of the glenohumeral joint is improved by strong muscles, which compensate for weak ligaments.

Surgical approach. Surgical reattachment of the labrum to the glenoid rim is necessary for recurrent dislocations. The procedure may be done through an open incision or by arthroscopy. Bone grafting may be needed to fix glenoid rim fractures or, on rare occasions, Hill-Sachs lesions (**Fig. 2-20**).

II. ARM

A. Anatomy

Flexion of the elbow is mainly made possible by the action of the biceps and brachialis muscles, which lie on the anterior side of the humerus (**Fig. 2-21**). These muscles are innervated by the musculocutaneous nerve. The brachial artery, the median and ulnar nerves cruise down on the medial side of the arm. On the posterior side of the shaft of the humerus rest the triceps muscle bellies, which provide extension of the elbow. The radial nerve innervates this group of muscles as it crosses just posterior to the distal third of the humerus.

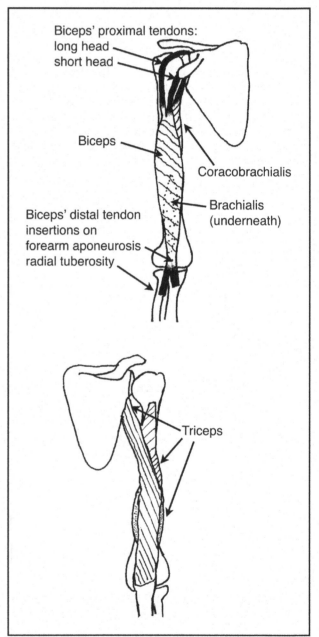

Fig. 2-21 Arm muscles.

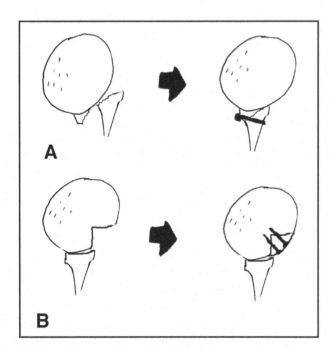

Fig. 2-20 Shoulder dislocation. A: Osseous Bankart treated with ORIF. **B:** Hill-Sachs lesion treated with bone grafting.

B. Approach

The approach mainly consists in testing the muscles that are anchored on the humerus. The most frequently injured muscle is the biceps, which can tear at its origin (long head of the biceps), or at its insertion at the bicipital tuberosity on the proximal radius. History of trauma will identify the cause for a fractured humerus.

C. Specific Problems

1. *Proximal biceps tendon rupture*

This problem is common in elderly patients and is often associated with chronic rotator cuff tears. It is also common in individuals involved in heavy manual labor.

Clinical Findings

Patients with chronic shoulder symptoms may feel a sudden sharp pain due to complete tearing of a degenerative long head of the biceps tendon. There is bulging of the biceps muscle in the bottom part of the arm due to loss of tension on the muscle. Muscle spasms may be present for a few weeks.

Treatment

Conservative approach. A conservative approach is usually reserved for elderly patients. It consists of ice application, NSAIDs, and rest. There is usually no severe loss of function besides mild weakness in flexion of the elbow.

Surgical approach. In younger individuals involved in physical labor or activities, fixing the tendon to the bicipital groove (*tenodesis*) will restore normal function and cosmesis (**Fig. 2-22**).

2. *Distal biceps tendon rupture*

This injury typically occurs in manual laborers after a strenuous effort while lifting a heavy load.

Clinical Findings

The main feature is proximal migration of the biceps muscle due to loss of its distal attachment. Palpation of the crease of the elbow (*antecubital fossa*) with absence of a cordlike structure (biceps tendon) is classic.

An MRI will reveal partial or complete tears of the biceps tendon. The extent of tendon retraction can also be evaluated.

Treatment

Conservative approach. A patient who consults 2 to 3 weeks after a distal biceps tendon tear may benefit from physiotherapy to improve residual strength and endurance.

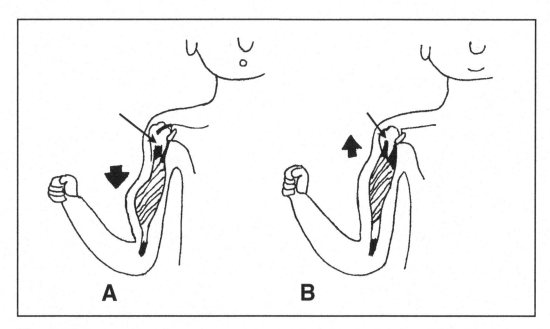

Fig. 2-22 Proximal biceps tendon rupture. A: Proximal biceps stump (thin arrow) retracted distally (thick arrow showing direction of retraction) with bulging of the biceps muscle. **B:** Surgical repair (thin arrow) and restoration of biceps muscle shape by pulling the muscle stump proximally (thick arrow).

Surgical approach. Surgery is considered as soon as possible to avoid retraction and scarring of the biceps muscle. It consists of reattaching the tendon to the biceps tuberosity of the radius (**Fig. 2-23**). Strengthening exercises begin after 3 months. Heavy labor is possible at 5-6 months post-op.

3. Humeral shaft fracture

Humeral shaft fractures are frequent in the elderly after a simple fall. In young individuals, a high energy trauma is required, such as in a motor vehicle accident (MVA).

Clinical Findings

This injury may cause a paralysis of the forearm extensor muscles (*CON lesion; c.f. Chap.1, section 3*). With a radial nerve injury, the patient cannot extend the wrist and fingers. The radial nerve is vulnerable with middle and distal third humeral shaft fractures. This is due to its close proximity to the bone, such that entrapment in the fracture site may occur. It is important to document if the nerve is intact or injured at the initial evaluation. A nerve injury present at the initial evaluation may signify that the nerve was bruised during the trauma and not necessarily squeezed between fracture fragments. A sudden paralysis of the forearm extensor muscles at the moment of splinting of the arm implies nerve entrapment.

Treatment

Conservative approach. Most humeral shaft fractures can be treated conservatively. The treatment consists of placing the arm in a plaster splint with the elbow flexed to 90 degrees. A sling can be provided for comfort (**Fig. 2-24**). Healing can take as long as 8 to 10 weeks. When radial nerve injury is present at the initial examination, monthly follow-up visits to monitor nerve recovery is required. Full recovery may take up to a year. Bracing of the forearm to keep the wrist and hand fingers extended will prevent contractures of the forearm muscles while awaiting recovery.

Surgical approach. Grossly displaced fractures, pathologic fractures, humeral fractures in polytraumatized patients (several other fractures), and bilateral humeral fractures are usually treated with ORIF or intramedullary nailing (**Fig. 2-24**). A radial nerve injury that appears while manipulating the arm for splinting implies nerve entrapment and warrants surgical exploration during ORIF.

III. ELBOW

A. Anatomy

The elbow is composed of three joints between the humerus, ulna, and radius (**Fig. 2-25**). The distal humerus articulates with the olecranon of the proximal ulna (*ulno-*

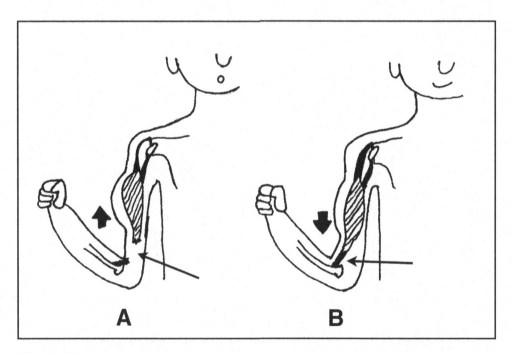

Fig. 2-23 Distal biceps tendon rupture. A: Distal biceps stump (thin arrow) retracted proximally (thick arrow) with bulging of the biceps muscle. **B:** Surgical repair (thin arrow) and restoration of biceps with bulging muscle shape by pulling the muscle stump distally (thick arrow).

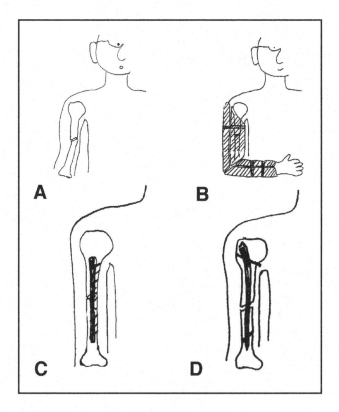

Fig. 2-24 Humeral shaft fracture. A: Mid-humeral shaft fracture. **B:** Fracture immobilization with a molded splint. **C:** Fracture ORIF. **D:** Intramedullary nailing.

humeral joint) and the radial head (*radio-capitellar joint*). Pronation and supination of the forearm is possible due to movement between the radial head and the ulna (*radio-ulnar joint*). On each side of the distal humerus are the collateral ligaments (**Fig. 2-26**). The bony prominences are called the *medial* and *lateral epicondyles,* where there are the Common Flexor Origin (CFO) and the Common Extensor Origin (CEO) of the forearm muscles.

The *olecranon bursa* is located posterior to the olecranon and allows smooth gliding of the overlying skin during motion. Anterior to the elbow joint is the *antecubital fossa.* The antecubital fossa contains the radial nerve, brachial artery and the median nerve. The ulnar nerve lies just behind the medial epicondyle posteriorly.

B. Approach

Ask questions about the onset, duration, localization, and type of pain. An acute pain may be due to a septic condition, whereas chronic pain may be an inflammatory articular condition (rheumatoid arthritis) or peri-articular (*epicondylitis*). Tingling or numbness locally or referred to the ulnar side of the hand may be due to compression or irritation of the ulnar nerve. Occupational inquiry is important since changes to the work environment or sports habits may help with the recovery.

The physical examination is summarized below:

1. Inspection: –skin lesion
                 –swelling
                 –deformity (valgus, varus, flexum)

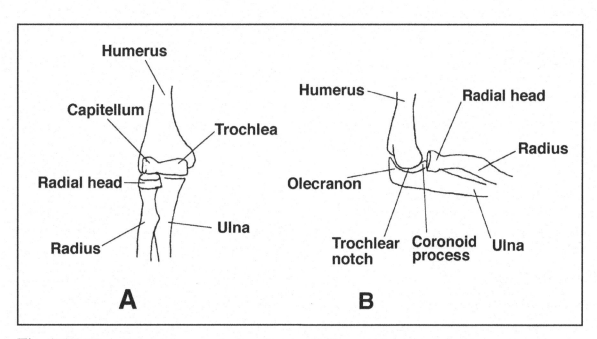

Fig. 2-25 Elbow joint anatomy. A: Anterior view. **B:** Lateral view.

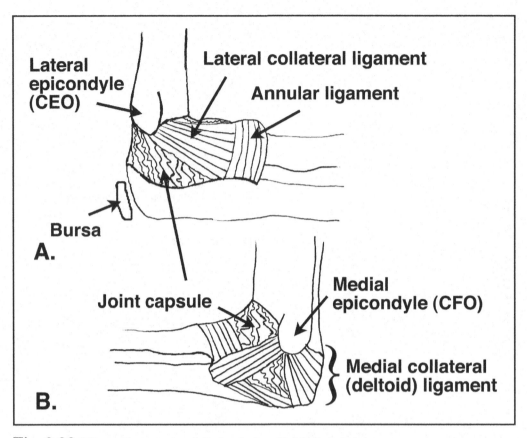

Fig. 2-26 Elbow ligaments. **A:** Lateral view. **B:** Medial view.

2. Range of motion (active): –extension/flexion
–supination/pronation

3. Palpation:
   i) Posterior part: –warmth
–swelling
–sensitivity
–nodules
   ii) Anterior part: –warmth
–swelling
–radial head
–sensitivity of epicondyles
with and without active
flexion and extension of the
wrist and fingers

4. Specific maneuvers: –valgus and varus stress to
test the collateral ligaments

C. Specific Problems

1. Tennis and golf elbow (epicondylitis)

Patients of 30 to 50 years of age practicing an activity involving repetitive movement of the forearm are at risk for medial and lateral epicondylitis. The extensor muscles of the forearm are active for the stabilization of the wrist, as for the backhand stroke in tennis (*tennis elbow*). The flexor muscles of the forearm are solicited for stabilizing the wrist during the forward swing in golf (*golfer's elbow*).

Clinical Findings

The pain is localized to the lateral epicondyle at the *common extensor origin (CEO)* or to the medial epicondyle at the *common flexor origin (CFO)*. To reproduce the pain, have the patient extend or flex the wrist against resistance. The pain might be so intense that no active resistance is possible.

Simple X-ray views of the elbow are usually normal. MRI may be useful to evaluate possible ligamentous or tendinous injuries of the elbow.

Treatment

Conservative approach. Most tendinitis can be treated by eliminating activities causing pain and adapting working conditions or sports techniques. NSAIDs, steroid infiltrations, physical therapy, and an epicondylar band over the forearm muscles to decrease force transmission to the tendons are useful. Return to regular activities should be progressive to prevent recurrence.

Surgical approach. Surgery is considered after failure of 6 to 12 months of conservative treatment. It consists of releasing the muscle group origin from the epicondyle.

2. Olecranon bursitis

Patients often present after a direct trauma or because of spontaneous local inflammation (i.e., gout).

Clinical Findings

The main finding is significant swelling of the soft tissues over the olecranon. Warmth, redness, and history of fever suggest possible infection of the bursa.

On a lateral radiograph of the elbow, prominence of soft tissues posterior to the olecranon can be seen, causing contour deformity.

Treatment

Conservative approach. For the first event, aspiration of the bursa is done using sterile technique. The liquid is usually serous and of a yellowish color. The elbow is then wrapped with an elastic bandage for 2 weeks. NSAIDs may be prescribed. If the bursitis recurs, the aspiration is repeated and 1 ml of corticosteroid (40 mg/ml) is injected. The arm is then immobilized in a splint for 2 weeks. The main objective is to prevent friction about the elbow and to reduce inflammation.

Surgical approach. Recurrent bursitis can be treated surgically by removal of the bursa (*bursectomy*). Infected bursitis is rarely successfully treated with antibiotics alone. After culture, debridement and irrigation of the wound, antibiotics are continued for 7 to 10 days.

3. Distal humeral fracture

Clinical Findings

The main clinical finding to rule out is loss of wrist extension due to radial nerve injury. Also, the obliquity and spiky nature of the fracture lines can cause small puncture wounds through the skin. These open fractures can be easily missed (*CON lesion; c.f. Chap.1, section 3*).

Treatment

Conservative approach. Non-displaced fractures are treated with a cast or a splint from the axilla to the wrist with 90 degrees of flexion at the elbow (**Fig. 2-27A-B**). The cast is removed after 6 weeks to start physical therapy. If the fracture has a complex pattern, then the arm can be put in a molded articulated brace for another

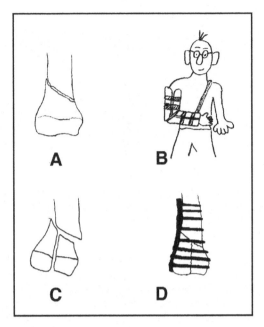

Fig. 2-27 Distal humeral fracture. A: Simple non-displaced distal humeral fracture. **B:** Conservative treatment with splinting. **C:** Displaced comminuted intra-articular distal humeral fracture. **D:** Surgical treatment with ORIF.

6 weeks to protect from twisting (rotational) stresses with the movement of the arm.

Surgical approach. Displaced fractures and severely comminuted fractures are treated surgically (**Fig. 2-27C-D**). Most fractures with radial nerve injury warrant surgical exploration due to the high incidence of nerve entrapment at this level.

4. Olecranon fracture

Olecranon fracture is usually caused by a direct fall on the elbow while trying to protect oneself when falling backwards.

Clinical Findings

The skin on the elbow is usually very thin and is easily perforated by bony fragments (*CON lesion; c.f. Chap.1, section 3*). An open fracture can easily be mistaken for an abrasion.

Simple AP and lateral X-ray views are diagnostic.

Treatment

Conservative approach. A non-displaced fracture can be treated with a full arm cast molded at 90 degrees of flexion. Close weekly follow-up is recommended for the first 3 weeks to pick up any displacement of the fragments during healing. Usually, 4 weeks of immobilization is sufficient. Physical therapy will restore the range of motion, but a residual deficit in elbow extension usually remains.

Surgical approach. An olecranon fracture is an intra-articular fracture, and any displacement of more than 2 mm requires ORIF or pinning (**Fig. 2-28**). Rigid fixation may not require additional splinting afterwards, and physical therapy can be started as soon as possible.

5. Radial head fracture

A radial head fracture is mainly caused by a sudden stress in valgus.

Clinical Findings

The pain is localized to the radial head on palpation. Pronation and supination of the forearm cause severe pain. Blockage can occur due to a displaced fragment. A xylocaine intra-articular injection can discriminate true mechanical blockage from loss of pro/supination simply due to pain.

Simple X-ray views of the elbow may not show a subtle, non-displaced fracture of the radial head. However, the presence of a joint effusion, seen as displacement of the anterior elbow fat pad (*sailboat sign*) should alert you to the possibility of a non-displaced radial head fracture (**Fig. 2-29**).

Treatment

Conservative approach. Non-displaced fractures are treated with sling immobilization for 3 weeks. Progres-

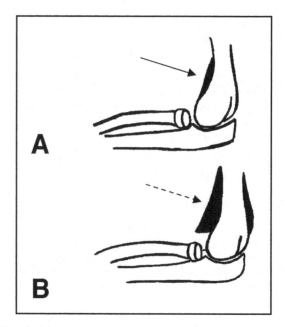

Fig. 2-29 Sailboat sign. A: Normal fat pad (straight line) appearance on X-ray lateral view. **B:** Displaced fat pad (dashed line) analogous to sail boat appearance.

sive motion is started thereafter. The patient must be informed of a likely loss of extension. Physical therapy is usually needed to regain near normal range of motion.

Surgical approach. Displaced fractures and fractures with mechanical blockage of pro/supination require surgery. The surgery may consist of ORIF or radial head resection if comminution is severe (**Fig. 2-30**).

6. Elbow dislocation

This injury occurs with hyperextension and torsion of the arm.

Clinical Findings

With this injury, the swelling around the elbow may be so impressive that the actual dislocation may be overlooked. If there is less swelling, the olecranon process is prominent posteriorly, which is a clear indicator of elbow dislocation.

Simple X-ray views may reveal a fracture of the coronoid process or the radial head. When a fracture is present in the context of an elbow dislocation, instability or redislocation of the elbow can occur after reduction.

Treatment

Conservative approach. Immediate reduction is mandatory. After mild sedation, push on the olecranon rather

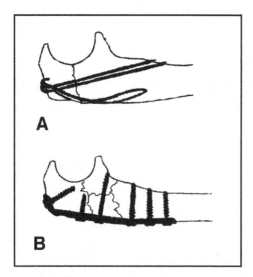

Fig. 2-28 Olecranon fracture ORIF. A: Stabilization of a simple fracture with K-wires and steel cable. **B:** Comminuted fracture stabilized with plate and screws.

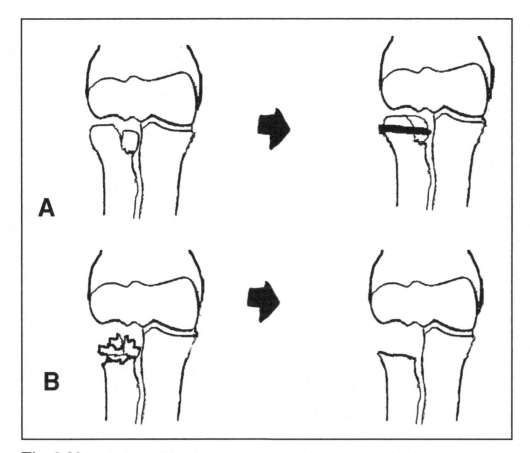

Fig. 2-30 Radial head fracture treatment. A: Anterior view of a simple radial head fracture treated with ORIF. **B:** Anterior view of a comminuted radial head fracture treated with radial head excision.

than pulling on the arm (**Fig. 2-31**). Physical therapy is started after keeping the elbow immobilized in a sling for 3 weeks. After the reduction, if the elbow redislocates with mild extension, it must then be immobilized in a cast for 6 weeks to allow the ligaments to heal and restore stability.

Surgical approach. Surgery is indicated when the elbow easily redislocates due to the presence of a fracture. ORIF of the fractures will restore stability. A cast is applied for 3 to 6 weeks, depending on surgeon preference, degree of stability, and rigidity of fixation.

IV. FOREARM

A. Anatomy

The bones of the forearm are the radius and ulna (**Fig. 2-32**). The distal radius articulates with the distal ulna to form the distal radioulnar joint (DRUJ). The wrist and finger extensor muscles, and the wrist supinator muscles lie on the dorsal side of the forearm. The innervation of these muscles is provided by the radial nerve. The wrist and finger flexor muscles, and the wrist

pronator muscles are on the volar (palmar) side of the forearm. Innervation of these muscles is provided by the ulnar and median nerves. The radial and ulnar arteries course on the volar side of the forearm. Both arteries can be palpated distally over their respective bones.

B. Approach

Ask questions about the onset, the type, and duration of pain. Injuries occur in the context of trauma (ski fall, roller blade injury, motor vehicle accident). A systematic approach though: 1—Inspection, 2—Palpation, 3—Range of motion of the joints above and below, and 4—Neurovascular exam of the upper limbs will reveal the likely cause of pain.

C. Specific Problems

1. Radial and ulnar fractures

Clinical Findings

Fractures of the radius and ulna can be associated with a compartment syndrome (*CON lesion; c.f. Chap.1,*

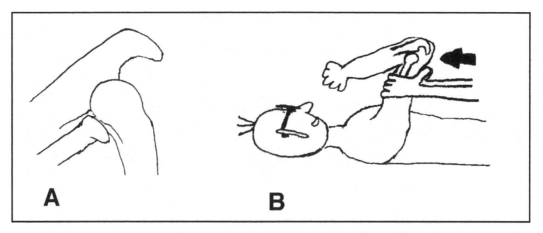

Fig. 2-31 Elbow dislocation. A: Lateral view of elbow dislocation. **B:** Reduction maneuver.

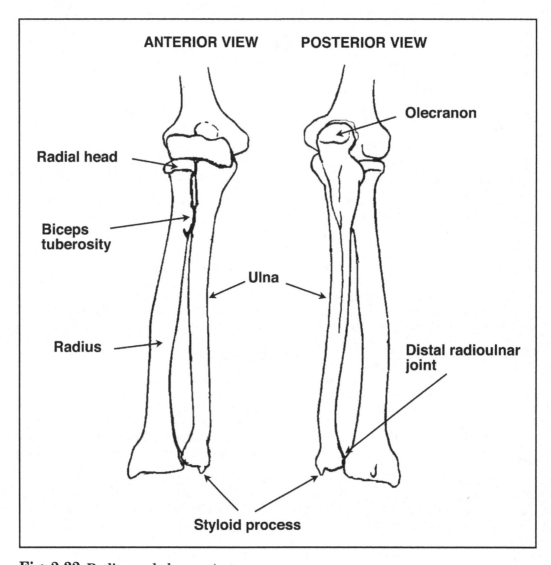

Fig. 2-32 Radius and ulna anatomy.

section 3) of the forearm. The clinician must keep in mind the 5 P's (pain, paresthesia, palpation of a hard compartment, paralysis, pallor/pulselessness) for clinical suspicion of a compartment syndrome.

Simple X-ray views of the forearm are diagnostic, but views of the elbow and wrist must be obtained to rule out associated joint dislocations.

Treatment

Conservative approach. For non-displaced fractures, use a full arm cast with 90 degrees of elbow flexion for 6 weeks. Prolonged immobilization may increase the risk of elbow stiffness.

Surgical approach. All displaced fractures are treated with ORIF. Surgical treatment allows quick mobilization of the arm (**Fig. 2-33**).

2. *Monteggia and Galeazzi fracture-dislocations*

At an Italian demonstration, the policeman Radii Galeazzi tried to hit a student named Ulna Monteggia with a night stick. Ulna Monteggia blocked the blow with his forearm and tripped Radii Galeazzi (the policeman), who fell on his outstretched hand. Both the student and the policeman were rushed to the hospital. The student, Ulna Monteggia, had to have surgery while Radii Galeazzi only got a cast. This story helps you to remember which bone is fractured, the mechanism of injury, and the treatment strategy in Galeazzi and Monteggia fracture-dislocations.

The Monteggia fracture-dislocation involves a fracture of the ulna and dislocation of the radial head (**Fig. 2-34A**). It is usually caused by a blow to the forearm when trying to protect oneself (just like the student Ulna Monteggia). A Galeazzi fracture dislocation (**Fig. 2-34C**) involves a fracture of the distal radius and dislocation of the distal ulna at the distal radio-ulnar joint due to a fall on an outstretched hand (just like the policeman Radii Galeazzi).

Clinical Findings

These particular injuries usually show significantly more deformity and swelling at the elbow (Monteggia) and the wrist (Galeazzi) than simple radial and ulnar fractures.

Simple X-rays views of the forearm, elbow, and wrist will reveal the type of injury.

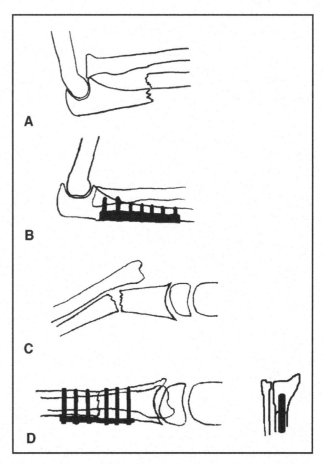

Fig. 2-34 Forearm fracture-dislocations. A: Monteggia type fracture. **B:** ORIF of the ulna with reduction of the radial head dislocation. **C:** Galeazzi type fracture. **D:** ORIF of the radius with reduction of the ulnar dislocation.

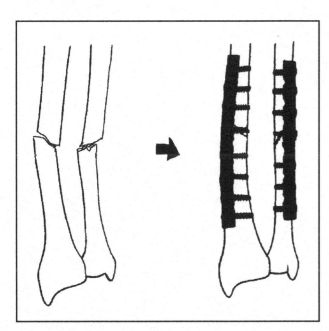

Fig. 2-33 ORIF of radial and ulnar fractures.

Treatment

Conservative approach. Satisfactory reduction after manual traction for a Monteggia fracture-dislocation is rarely achieved.

Galeazzi fracture-dislocation can be successfully treated conservatively. After reduction, a full arm cast with 90 degrees of elbow flexion is needed. The cast should extend over the wrist. The forearm is rotated in the best possible position (pronated, supinated, or neutral) to maintain the reduction of the distal radio-ulnar joint.

Surgical approach. A Monteggia fracture-dislocation is usually treated with ORIF of the ulna and reduction of the radial head (**Fig. 2-34B**). The arm is kept in a splint for 4 to 6 weeks.

A Galeazzi fracture-dislocation can be treated with ORIF of the radius only (**Fig. 2-34D**) or with pinning of the distal radio-ulnar joint if it is too unstable. The forearm is kept in a cast for 4 to 6 weeks.

3. *Distal radial and ulnar fractures*

Most fractures occur with a fall on an outstretched hand with the wrist in hyperextension. These fractures are predominantly seen in the elderly due to osteoporosis. Several types of fracture may occur at the distal radius (**Fig. 2-35**).

a. Colles' fracture

This injury is an extra-articular fracture of the distal radius with dorsal displacement of the distal fragment with the apex palmar angulation. On the lateral radiograph, the wrist takes on the appearance of a dinner fork (*dinner fork deformity*). The distal fragment is often impacted into the proximal one, which gives rise to shortening of the radius. Half of patients with a *Colles' fracture* also have a fracture of the ulnar styloid.

Abraham Colles (1773-1843) was the greatest teacher of surgery of the 19th century in Dublin School of Medicine.

b. Smith's fracture

Smith's fracture is intra-articular fracture of the palmar lip of the distal radius.

Robert William Smith (1807-1873) became the professor of surgery at Trinity College in Dublin, succeeding Colles, upon whom he performed the autopsy.

c. Barton's fracture

A *Barton fracture* is an intra-articular fracture of the dorsal lip of the distal radius.

John Rhea Barton (1794-1871) was an American surgeon from Lancaster, Pennsylvania.

Clinical Findings

Median nerve compression (*CON lesion; c.f. Chap.1, section 3*) can occur with significant fracture displace-

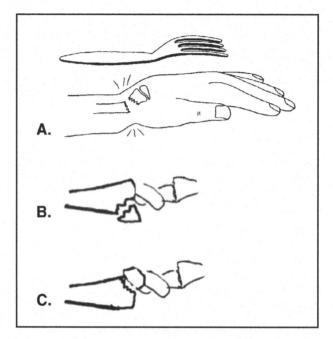

Fig. 2-35 Types of distal radial fracture. Lateral views. **A:** Colles' type is an extra-articular fracture with dorsal angulation. The apparent deformation is also known as "dinner fork deformity". **B:** Smith's type is an intra-articular fracture with displacement of the palmar articular surface. **C:** Barton's type is an intra-articular fracture with displacement of the dorsal articular surface.

ment. This causes paresthesia in the thumb, index, and middle fingers.

Simple AP and lateral views are sufficient. Oblique views may be obtained in equivocal cases. A scaphoid fracture can be associated with a distal radius fracture and must be ruled out.

Treatment

Conservative approach. Non-displaced distal radius fractures are treated with cast immobilization for 6 weeks. Slightly displaced fractures can be reduced under local anesthesia. After inserting the syringe needle directly into the fracture line, the syringe piston is pulled back. Using blood appearing in the syringe as a sign that the needle is in the hematoma of the fracture, then the Lidocaine is injected (*hematoma block*) to provide enough relief for the reduction. The cast is applied and molded to maintain the reduction. The patient must be followed weekly with X-rays to assess for any displacement that might occur in the cast.

Surgical approach. Displaced or comminuted fractures are treated with percutaneous pinning with wires, ORIF, or an external fixator (**Fig. 2-36**). A combination

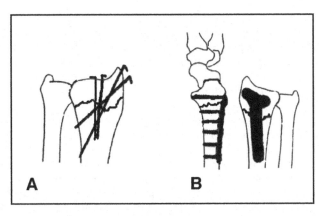

Fig. 2-36 Distal radius fracture. A: ORIF with K-wire. **B:** ORIF with plate and screws.

of these techniques may be used. An intra-articular fracture with more than a 2 mm step-off deformity at the cartilaginous surface is usually treated with ORIF, since a perfect reduction is required.

V. WRIST AND HAND

A. Anatomy

The carpal bones are in a two-row configuration (**Fig. 2-37**). The scaphoid and lunate bones are part of the proximal carpal row. The carpal bones are linked to one another with strong ligaments. They articulate by gliding against one another in a synchronized fashion. The *flexor retinaculum* is palmar to the carpal bones

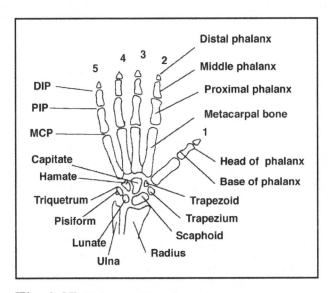

Fig. 2-37 Wrist and hand anatomy.

and defines the carpal tunnel. The carpal tunnel is a finite space that contains the flexor tendons of the hand and the median nerve.

The hand consists of the metacarpal bones, which articulate with the carpal bones. The metacarpal bones articulate with the phalanges distally (**Fig. 2-37**). The movement at metacarpophalangeal (MCP), and interphalangeal (IP) joints is made possible by the action of the flexor tendons passing through tendon sheaths and pulleys. The median nerve innervates the flexor muscles of the thumb, index finger, and half of the long finger. It also provides sensitivity to the palmar side of these fingers. The ulnar nerve innervates the flexor muscles of the 5th, 4th and half of the long fingers. It also provides sensitivity to the palmar side of these fingers. The radial nerve innervates the extensor muscles of all the fingers and provides sensitivity to the dorsum of the hand. The extensor tendons glide under the *extensor retinaculum* of the wrist by going through 6 tube-like structures known as the extensor compartments up to the base of the distal phalanx of each finger.

B. Approach

Ask about the precise location of the pain. A diffusely painful wrist may represent a synovitis. Pain at the base of the thumb may involve extensor tendons (*de Quervain tenosynovitis*) or carpometacarpal arthritis. Pain with tingling sensation on the palmar side on the hand suggests a median or cubital nerve neuropathy. The onset and trigger of pain help distinguish between an inflammatory and a mechanical condition. History of trauma or presence of systemic symptoms may greatly help to pinpoint the diagnosis.

The physical examination is summarized below:

1. Inspection:
    i) dorsal aspect: –swelling
                        –deformation
                        –muscular atrophy
    ii) palmar aspect: –swelling
                        –muscular atrophy
                        –skin lesion

2. Palpation: –warmth
                 –for pain at wrist, MP, PIP, DIP joints

3. Range of motion: –active and passive by making a fist and extending the fingers completely

4. Specific maneuvers: –evaluate grip strength with grip dynamometer (Newton)
                          –upper limb reflexes
                          –Phalen (**Fig. 2-38**) and Tinel (**Fig. 2-39**) signs.

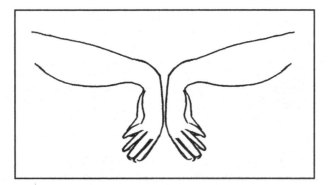

Fig. 2-38 Phalen test. The patient flexes both wrists against one another and holds this position for one minute. In the presence of a carpal tunnel syndrome, the numbness in the median nerve territory can be reproduced.

C. Specific Problems

1. Carpal tunnel syndrome

Carpal tunnel syndrome is a median nerve neuropathy resulting from increased pressure within the carpal tunnel. It is usually idiopathic. However, it can also occur with hormonal imbalance, such as in pregnancy, thyroid disorders, and diabetes.

Clinical Findings

Thumb, index, and long finger numbness at night is pathognomonic of carpal tunnel syndrome. Patients will often have decreased 2 point sensory discrimination in the median nerve territory. Patients with chronic carpal tunnel syndrome may have thenar eminence atrophy and weakness of thumb opposition. If there is marked swelling of the wrist, there may be an underlying inflammatory disorder.

The *Tinel sign* may be positive: median nerve percussion at the wrist level reproduces the symptoms. The *Phalen sign* may also be positive: maintained passive flexion of the wrist increases nerve compression and reproduces the symptoms in less than one minute.

EMG and nerve conduction velocity studies may help with the diagnosis. Other tests such as inflammatory serology, glycemia, and thyroid tests may be indicated.

Treatment

Conservative approach. Semi-rigid immobilization with wrist splints at night can help decrease the symptoms by preventing wrist flexion during sleep. NSAIDs and steroid infiltration may be used when there is tenosynovitis of the wrist.

Surgical approach. Patients with symptoms that do not respond to conservative therapy, those with chronic signs of carpal tunnel syndrome or EMG findings, may require surgical release of the flexor retinaculum.

2. Kienböck's Disease

Kienböck's disease is avascular necrosis of the lunate. It mostly affects the dominant hand. The history for trauma (hyperextension injury) is positive in 75% of patients.

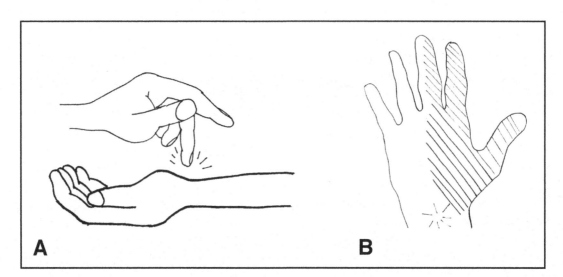

Fig. 2-39 Tinel sign. A: This sign is performed by tapping on the wrist of the patient to trigger tingling and numbness in the median nerve territory. **B:** Palmar view of the hand with median nerve territory highlighted (shaded area).

Clinical Findings

There is pinpoint tenderness over the lunate. The pain may be present up to 18 months before radiological signs. MRI may be obtained for early diagnosis.

An AP X-ray view may show an ulna that is shorter than the radius at the wrist level (*ulnar minus variance*), which may predispose patients to Kienböck's disease. The lunate may be whiter than other bones (indicating sclerosis). It eventually collapses, and in advanced disease, there is associated arthritis.

Treatment

Conservative approach. Splinting of the wrist may help with the symptoms but has no real impact on the evolution of the disease.

Surgical approach. When the ulna appears to be much shorter than the radius (ulnar minus variance), surgical intervention may be done to attempt to decrease the forces transmitted to the lunate by shortening the radius or lengthening the ulna. In more advanced disease, the surgeon can do a partial fusion with adjacent carpal bones, or complete fusion of the carpal bones with the radius (*wrist arthrodesis*). Elderly individuals or people with low demand activities can have the proximal row of carpal bones resected (*carpectomy*) to relieve the pain.

3. *De Quervain tenosynovitis*

De Quervain tenosynovitis is an inflammation of the tendons that glide through the first extensor compartment, which contains the abductor pollicis longus (APL) and the extensor pollicis brevis (EPB) and glide under the extensor retinaculum.

Clinical Findings

De Quervain tenosynovitis manifests itself by progressive pain with mobilization of the thumb, especially extension and abduction. The pain is localized to the first extensor tendon compartment. Crepitation may be present. The *Finkelstein test* is positive. This test involves having the patient flex the thumb into the palm of the hand. Upon ulnar deviation of the wrist, the pain is reproduced.

Treatment

Conservative approach. NSAIDs or steroid infiltration within the first extensor compartment can be tried. If the pain persists, immobilization of the thumb for 4-6 weeks with a splint or a thumb "spica" (*Latin spicatus, forming a spike*) cast, which extends up to the thumb finger nail.

Surgical approach. For the persistent or recurrent De Quervain tenosynovitis, surgery can be done to open the first extensor tendon compartment to release the tendons, and to remove any inflammatory synovium (*synovectomy*).

4. *Dupuytren contracture*

Dupuytren contracture is a disease of the fascia of the hand and was described by Baron Guillaume Dupuytren (1777-1835). He was the ultimate workaholic and became one of the richest doctors of his time, seeing up to 10,000 patients a year.

Clinical Findings

With palpation, the contractures of palmar fascia (cords) can be felt in the palm of the hand. The affected fingers can eventually be drawn into palmar flexion by the contracture of the cords so that they cannot be fully extended. All the digits, including the thumb, can be affected, but most commonly, the ring and little fingers are involved. It can be associated with plantar fascia contracture (*Lederhosen's*) or penile involvement (*Peyronie's*).

Treatment

Conservative approach. No proven treatment has been shown to reverse the disease.

Surgical approach. Surgical excision of all diseased cords (*fasciectomy*) can be successful.

5. *Trigger finger (stenosing flexor tenosynovitis)*

Trigger finger is an inflammation of a flexor tendon preventing easy gliding of the tendon through the hand pulleys. This results in an abrupt flexion of the finger much like the sudden motion of pulling on a trigger. Extension of the finger is also abrupt or totally prevented in more severe cases.

Clinical Findings

The classical clinical findings of a trigger finger are pain over the A1 pulley (a fibrous structure located at the MCP joint through which the flexor tendons pass) and intermittent blockage of flexion and extension of the finger due to the difficult passage of the inflamed tendon through the unyielding pulley.

Treatment

Conservative approach. A steroid infiltration into the affected tendon's sheath can decrease symptoms in 90% of cases. Splinting of the finger can help decrease the inflammation along the tendon and eventually allow gliding through the pulley.

Surgical approach. Surgical release of the A1 flexor pulley will allow the inflamed tendon to go through and will relieve the symptoms.

6. Scaphoid fracture

Scaphoid fractures commonly occur in young individuals following a fall on an outstretched hand (*FOOSH*). The scaphoid bone has a precarious vascular supply. Damage to its blood supply can cause avascular necrosis of the proximal fragment and nonunion. These conditions can lead to degenerative changes and chronic wrist pain.

Clinical Findings

A classic sign for a scaphoid fracture is tenderness or pain on palpation over the anatomical "*snuff box*". This is a depression on the back of the hand, just beneath the thumb, that is formed by three extensor tendons. When sniffing tobacco (snuff) was popular, this small compartment could be used as a place to hold the tobacco.

There is also painful and limited wrist dorsiflexion. Scaphoid fractures can be associated with a tear of the ligament between the scaphoid and lunate. This may lead to an increased scapholunate interval (greater than 5 mm) and wrist instability. There is also an increased risk of osteonecrosis of the proximal pole of the scaphoid bone.

If a scaphoid fracture is clinically suspected, dedicated scaphoid X-rays should be obtained in addition to simple AP and lateral views of the wrist. If the X-rays are negative immediately following the trauma, a scaphoid fracture may be present but not yet visible. Follow-up X-rays, CT, or MRI may reveal an occult fracture.

Treatment

Conservative approach. Non-displaced scaphoid fractures are treated with a thumb spica cast, which extends to the base of the thumb nail (**Fig. 2-40A**). The cast is kept on for a minimum of 12 weeks. If the fracture heals, there should be no pain over the anatomical snuff box upon cast removal. Cast treatment should be applied for up to 2 weeks if such a fracture is suspected, and X-rays are repeated weekly for diagnosis. If no fracture line is visible after 2 weeks, then the cast is removed.

Surgical approach. Displaced fractures of more than 2 mm are treated with ORIF (**Fig. 2-40B**). Non-united fractures which are not displaced can be treated with a percutaneous screw. Displaced non-united fractures need ORIF and bone grafting.

7. Peri-lunate and lunate dislocations

Peri-lunate dislocation occurs when the capitate bone dislocates dorsally relative to the lunate (**Fig. 2-41**). A lunate dislocation is when the lunate bone dislocates volar relative to the radius. The mechanism of injury is forced dorsiflexion of the wrist.

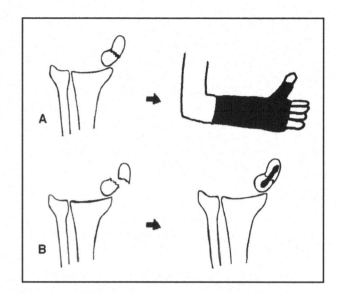

Fig. 2-40 Scaphoid fracture. A: Non-displaced scaphoid fracture is treated conservatively with forearm cast up to the base of the thumb. **B:** Displaced scaphoid fracture treated with ORIF.

Clinical Findings

The wrist is swollen with extreme pain upon mild mobilization. It is important not to miss associated median nerve compression (*CON lesion; c.f. Chap.1, section 3*), which is a medical emergency.

The carpal dislocation is best seen on the lateral view.

Treatment

Conservative approach. Peri-lunate and lunate dislocations cannot be treated conservatively.

Surgical approach. Reduction of the lunate bone is difficult and most successfully done in the operating

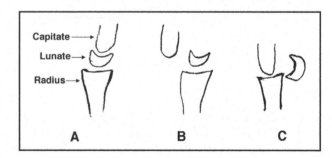

Fig. 2-41 Carpal dislocations. A: Normal carpal alignment. **B:** Peri-lunate dislocation with the capitate no longer in contact with the lunate. **C:** Lunate dislocation with the lunate off its normal position between the distal radius and the capitate.

room. If the scapho-lunate ligament appears intact during open reduction, consider cast immobilization for 6 to 8 weeks. A torn scapholunate ligament mandates pinning with or without ligament reconstruction.

8. *First metacarpal base fracture*

Once upon a time, the great singer Tony Bennett was being driven by his chauffeur Rolando. All of a sudden, the engine stalled and they had to hitchhike home. Although both of them had sore thumbs, Rolando's thumb hurt the most because he did most of the hitchhiking. This story can help you remember that Bennett's and Rolando's fractures are located at the base of the first metacarpal bone and that Rolando's fracture is worse. Fractures of the first metacarpal base result from axial forces on a flexed metacarpal.

Clinical Findings

The pain and swelling at the base of the first metacarpal can be impressive.

Simple X-ray views of the hand with added magnified views of the first metacarpal base are diagnostic (**Fig. 2-42**). A Bennett's fracture is a single intra-articular fracture of the base of the first metacarpal bone. The larger radial fragment is dislocated dorsally and radially by the abductor pollicis longus muscle. Bennett's fracture must be distinguished from extra-articular fractures. The Rolando fracture is a comminuted intra-articular fracture of the base of the first metacarpal bone. Rolando's fracture has a worse prognosis than the Bennett's fracture.

Treatment

Conservative approach. Non-displaced fractures are treated with a thumb spica cast.

Surgical approach. A displaced fracture must be reduced by traction and stabilization, usually with percu-

taneous pinning. A fracture with a fragment > 15% of the articular surface is treated with ORIF.

9. *Skier's thumb (ulnar collateral ligament injury)*

The *skier's thumb* injury results from forced abduction of the first metacarpo-phalangeal joint. This injury often occurs after a fall while holding a ski pole (**Fig. 2-43**).

Clinical Findings

There is pain on palpation over the ulnar collateral ligament (UCL) of the MCP joint of the thumb. Instability of the joint may result from avulsion of the base of the proximal phalanx by the UCL.

On simple X-ray views of the thumb, a bony avulsion of the base of the proximal phalanx may be visible. Interposition of the adductor pollicis muscle aponeurosis between this fragment and the base of the phalanx (*Stener lesion*) may prevent healing (**Fig. 2-44**). Stener doesn't necessarily have to be associated with a fracture. It can be due to only a ligament tear. MRI is diagnostic.

Treatment

Conservative approach. Incomplete collateral ligament tears can be treated with a thumb spica cast for 6 weeks followed by protective splinting. Pain may last for many months.

Surgical approach. If the bony fragment is displaced, a surgical reinsertion (ORIF) is indicated to restore

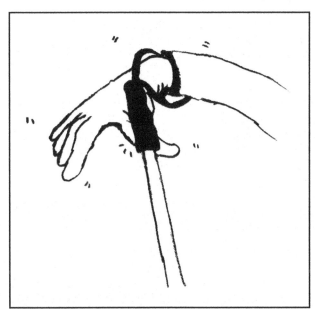

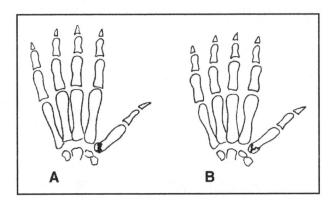

Fig. 2-42 First metacarpal base fracture.
A: Bennett's fracture. **B:** Rolando's fracture.

Fig. 2-43 Skier's thumb. The thumb is trapped behind the ski pole and forced into radial deviation.

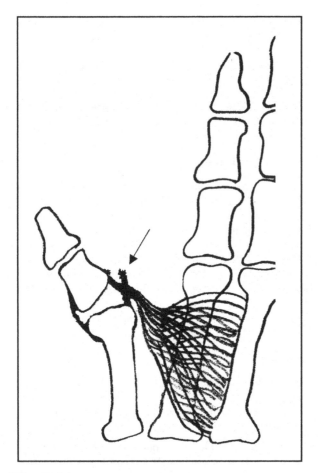

Fig. 2-44 Skier's thumb. Lesion of the ulnar collateral ligament (black arrow) at the thumb MP joint. A Stener lesion occurs when the ligament is prevented from healing to the base of the phalanx due to interposition of the thumb adductor tendon.

stability. A Stener lesion is treated surgically to remove the interposed structure and repair the UCL.

10. Boxer's fracture (fourth or fifth metacarpal neck fracture)

A metacarpal neck fracture usually results from strong axial force (like from a punch to a hard surface) (**Fig. 2-45**).

Clinical Findings

Look for a puncture wound (*CON lesion; c.f. Chap.1, section 3*) caused by the teeth of the opponent. Displacement of the distal metacarpal fragment can produce decreased extension or malrotation of the affected finger and prevent proper bending.

Simple X-ray views of the hand will show the extent of displacement.

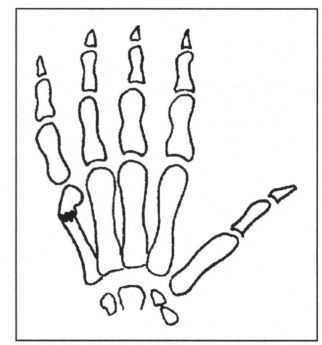

Fig. 2-45 Fifth metacarpal neck fracture (boxer's fracture).

Treatment

Conservative approach. Reduction is done under local anesthesia with the fifth finger in flexion (*Jahss maneuver*). The hand is splinted in the "hamburger" position (like holding a hamburger with one hand), also referred to as the "safe position" to immobilize the metacarpophalangeal joints. In this position, the MCP collateral ligaments are maximally stretched to minimize contracture during immobilization. The small finger may tolerate angulation of the head up to 40 degrees because of greater metacarpal mobility. If the skin was cut by a tooth, then antibiotic prophylaxis with penicillin is given for a week.

Surgical approach. Severe angulation must be reduced and stabilized with pinning or ORIF. A puncture wound from the opponent's teeth can inseminate the joint with germs from the oral flora and cause septic arthritis. To prevent infection of the joint, it is recommended to do an open debridement, irrigation, and prophylactic antibiotics for a week (Ancef 1 g IV q8h for 24 hours and Keflex 500 mg QID by mouth for 7 days).

11. Distal phalanx fractures

a. *Mallet (baseball) finger*

Mallet finger is a condition in which the DIP joint of a finger bends but will not straighten by itself due to rupture of the extensor tendon (**Fig. 2-46**). This may be associated with a fracture of the base of the distal phalanx.

b. Jersey finger

The *jersey finger* is a condition in which the DIP joint of a finger extends but will not flex by itself due to rupture or avulsion of the flexor digitorum profundus (**Fig. 2-47**). This kind of injury usually occurs from grabbing a jersey during a football tackle.

Clinical Findings

For the mallet finger, there is a flexed posture of the DIP joint. The mallet and jersey fingers are conditions possibly caused by a tendon rupture, a tendon laceration, or a partial intra-articular fracture of the distal phalanx.

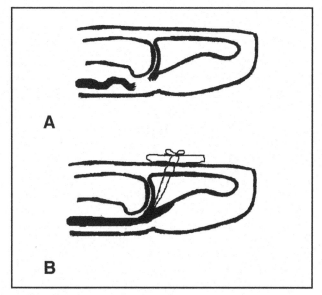

Fig. 2-47 Jersey finger. A: Flexor digitorum profundus tendon avulsion (thick black line) from distal phalanx. **B:** Tendon repair with pull-through suture (thin black line with a bow).

Simple X-rays of the involved finger will rule out a phalanx fracture.

Treatment

Conservative approach. The treatment for a mallet finger is continual splinting of the distal inter-phalangeal joint in extension for 6 to 8 weeks. There is no conservative approach for a jersey finger.

Surgical approach. A displaced intra-articular mallet fracture is treated with closed or open reduction with pinning. A jersey finger requires surgery to reattach the FDP tendon to the distal phalanx. The tendon can be repaired with a pull-through suture (**Fig. 2-47**) and splinting for 6 weeks.

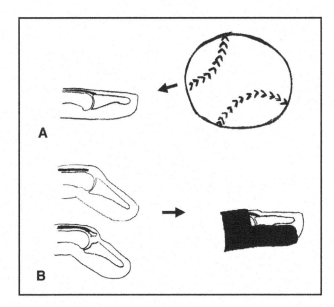

Fig. 2-46 Mallet (baseball) finger. A: Normal fingertip hit by a baseball. **B:** Tendon avulsion and bony avulsion mallet finger treated with a splint.

CHAPTER 3. LOWER LIMB

I. HIP

A. Anatomy

Imagine yourself in the days of the French Revolution when the Queen Femora is head of state (**Fig. 3-1**). Indeed, our Queen Femora (with her funky hat!) is somehow analogous to the hip joint, which is composed of the femoral head and the pelvic acetabulum. The neck of the femur is analogous to Queen Femora's neck with respect to vital blood vessels bringing blood flow to the head. Queen Femora is surrounded by many servants to help her move around, just as the hip joint is surrounded by numerous muscles to provide flexion (iliopsoas and rectus femoris muscles), extension (hamstrings and gluteus muscles), external rotation (short external rotator muscles), internal rotation and adduction (internal obturator and adductor muscles).

B. Approach

The clinician must differentiate articular, periarticular (trochanteric bursa or ischiopubic bones), or referred pain (originating from lower back and sacrum). Ask about age, pain triggering factors, maximal pain localization.

Pain present from infancy or appearing before 40 years of age signals a congenital pathology (hip dysplasia). Pain appearing after 60 years is most likely from degenerative disease (osteoarthritis). Pain from degenerative disease of the hip joint can also be referred to the knee and is also mechanical in nature (onset with weight bearing). Sudden inguinal pain is more likely with a traumatic event or sepsis. Precise pain localization over the greater trochanter strongly suggests bursitis.

With the patient standing:

1. Inspection:
   i) *Antalgic gait* (the patient will lean over the affected hip to bring the center of gravity over the joint to avoid a painful contraction of the hip abductors).
   ii) *Trendelenburg gait* (upon weight bearing over the painful hip, the pelvis and trunk will fall on the healthy side due to weak hip abductors.
   iii) standing position: –*scoliosis*
   –*pelvis asymmetry*
   –marked lumbar *lordosis* (*hyperlordosis*)

2. Specific maneuvers:
   i) Trendelenburg sign (**Fig. 3-2**)

With the patient lying down:

1. Inspection: –skin lesion
   –deformity
   –flexum (stiff hip with the knee raised off the table)
   –lower limb shortening

2. Palpation: –greater trochanter
   –ischial tuberosities
   –pubis

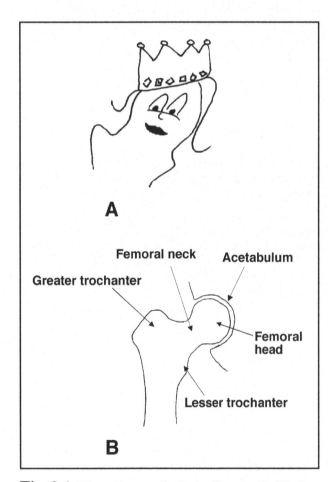

Fig. 3-1 Hip anatomy. A: Queen Femora. **B:** AP view of the hip joint.

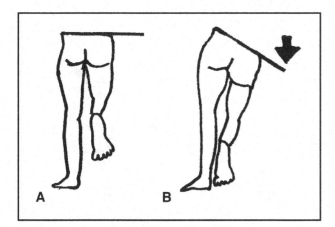

Fig. 3-2 Trendelenburg sign. A: Normal posture when lifting one foot off the floor with appropriate contraction of the abductors of the hip of the standing leg. **B:** Dropping of the pelvis due to weak abductors of the hip of the standing leg.

3. Range of motion (active /passive):
   –flexion, internal rotation, external rotation, abd/adduction

4. Specific maneuvers (**Fig. 3-3**):
   i) Thomas maneuver
   ii) FABER maneuver

C. Specific Problems

1. Trochanteric bursitis

Clinical Findings

The pain is localized to the lateral side of the hip just over the greater trochanter. It is reproduced by walking or by direct pressure over the greater trochanter.

X-rays are unremarkable.

Treatment

Conservative approach. The most successful therapy is rest with NSAIDs. A steroid infiltration can be performed for persistent or recurrent cases.

Surgical approach. Surgery is indicated after a failed conservative approach. It consists of resection of the bursa.

2. Hip fracture

Imagine that the revolutionaries decided to catch and drag Queen Femora to a famous and hip joint. Unfortunately for her, she was not the rave of the party. A guillotine was awaiting (**Fig. 3-4**). This dramatic story

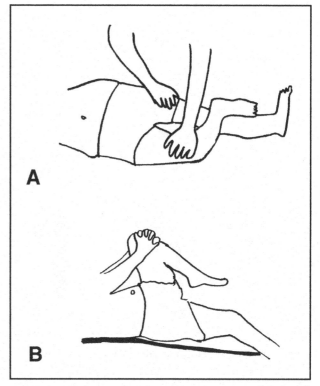

Fig. 3-3 Hip maneuvers. A: FABER also means flexion, abduction, external rotation. A positive FABER indicates a painful hip joint. **B:** A positive Thomas maneuver is present when the patient flexes the healthy hip by holding the knee close to the belly and the leg of the affected hip cannot lie flat against the exam table indicating contracture and lack of mobility.

summarizes the fact that losing her head brought a collapsed state. Interestingly, the hip can behave in much the same way.

Hip fractures are common in elderly people, particularly in women, who are more prone to developing osteoporosis.

Clinical Findings

The pain of a hip fracture is classically felt in the groin area. With the patient supine, the affected limb often lies in external rotation and there may be some apparent shortening.

Simple X-ray views of the hip are sufficient.

A femoral neck fracture may disrupt the blood supply to the femoral head. This may lead to the collapse of the femoral head from avascular necrosis (AVN). This is analogous to our famous Queen Femora, whose broken neck led to collapse of the head of state.

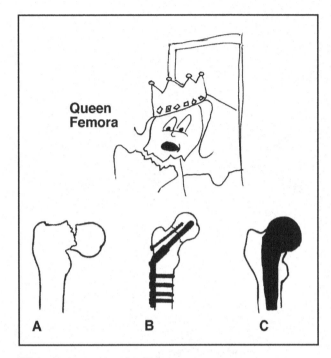

Fig. 3-4 Queen Femora with a neck fracture.
A: Displaced femoral neck fracture. **B:** ORIF with
screw and DHS. **C.** Femoral head replacement with
prosthesis.

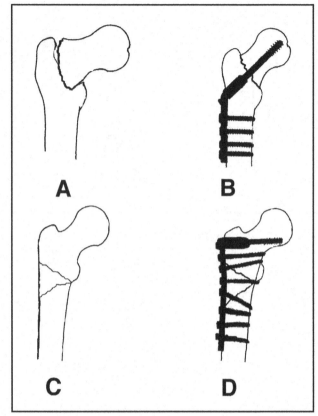

**Fig. 3-5 Intertrochanteric and subtrochanteric
hip fracture. A:** Displaced intertrochanteric fracture.
B: ORIF with DHS. **C:** Non-displaced subtrochanteric
fracture. **D:** ORIF with DHS.

Treatment

In the ER, a cutaneous traction of 5 lbs can be in-
stalled on the affected limb to provide alignment and
comfort. Patients with hip fractures have a high risk of
deep venous thrombosis (DVT). Antithrombotic prophylaxis, such as subcutaneous heparin, is indicated.

Conservative approach. This approach is usually reserved for extremely debilitated patients with other medical conditions that prevent surgery. It consists of analgesia
and progressive mobilization as tolerated by the patient.
This approach is prone to complications (decubitus ulcers,
pneumonia, DVT) due to prolonged bed rest.

Surgical approach. A hip fracture can be stabilized
by ORIF with 3 percutaneous screws when minimally
displaced. Greater displacement can be stabilized with
a dynamic hip screw (DHS) or with replacement of
the femoral head with a prosthesis, which allows for
quicker recovery (**Fig. 3-4**). The greater the displacement, the greater the risk of collapse of the femoral
head due to an avascular necrosis (AVN). Displaced
intertrochanteric and subtrochanteric fractures are
stabilized with a dynamic hip screw (DHS) (**Fig. 3-5**).
In younger individuals (<55 years old), an attempt at
ORIF must be considered since prostheses have a lim-

ited longevity, and revision surgery would be inevitable
in the long run.

3. Hip dislocation

Imagine Queen Femora "hip-hop" dancing in that famous and hip joint. She dances so hard that her head
slips out of her crown. This is analogous to a hip dislocation in which the hip "pops" out of the acetabulum
(**Fig. 3-6**). This problem occurs mainly in young adults
involved in motor vehicle accidents (MVA).

Clinical Findings

The affected limb is usually shorter, with severe pain
upon mobilization. Motor weakness or hypoesthesia in
the sciatic nerve territory (*CON lesion; c.f. Chap.1, section 3*), which is behind the thigh and all around the leg
and foot, is associated with posterior dislocation. Compression of the femoral artery and nerve is associated
with the rare anterior dislocation.

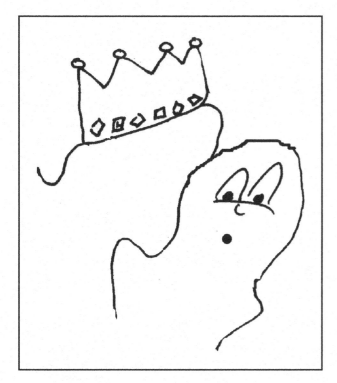

Fig. 3-6 Hip pops.

Simple X-ray views of the pelvis and AP and lateral views of the involved hip are necessary. A CT scan is the best exam to further evaluate associated fractures and is useful for planning the treatment.

Treatment

Conservative approach. A closed reduction of the femoral head can be done by manipulation and manual traction under general anesthesia. A control CT scan post-reduction is warranted to rule out loose bony fragments in the joint.

Surgical approach. Open reduction is rarely necessary. The indication would be a non-reducible dislocation due to interposed soft tissues. A dislocation with an associated fracture of the acetabular rim may require ORIF to restore stability.

II. THIGH

A. Anatomy

The main muscle groups at the thigh level are the quadriceps and the hamstrings. These muscles are responsible for the motion of the knee. The femoral nerve supplies the quadriceps muscle, and the sciatic nerve supplies the hamstrings while cruising straight down the back of the leg.

B. Approach

Assess the function of the quadriceps and hamstring muscles, and the integrity of the femur. A systematic approach with inspection, palpation, and analysis of the range of motion of the joints above and below will reveal most possible injuries to the thigh. A compartment syndrome within the thigh muscle compartments is rare but possible since a femoral fracture can bleed a lot. The clinician should be alert for the 5 P's (pain, paresthesia, paralysis, palpation of a hard compartment, pallor/paralysis) that may raise suspicion of a compartment syndrome.

C. Specific Problems

1. Femoral shaft fracture

All femur fractures in healthy adults occur after a violent trauma. They are often associated with other fractures.

Clinical Findings

A femoral fracture can cause significant bleeding (*CON lesion; c.f. Chap.1, section 3*) in the thigh, such that the patient's hemodynamics can be disturbed. Compartment syndrome within the thigh muscles is possible.

Simple X-ray views of the femur are diagnostic. Due to the usual high-energy trauma involved in femoral shaft fractures, close attention must be paid to the femoral neck to rule out an associated femoral neck fracture.

Treatment

In the emergency room. A femoral fracture is hard to immobilize. A skin traction applied on the leg or a Thomas splint, which gets its support from the ischium, can provide temporary immobilization to decrease the pain and facilitate the patient's transport to radiology.

Conservative approach. A critically ill patient who cannot undergo an operation may be treated with skeletal traction. Due to the prolonged bed rest, this approach is prone to complications, such as pressure sores (decubitus ulcers), DVT, and pneumonia.

Surgical approach. The vast majority of femoral fractures are treated surgically. The most frequently used technique is intra-medullar nailing (**Fig. 3-7**). ORIF with plate and screws is reserved for very proximal and distal fractures not amenable to nailing, or for severely comminuted fractures.

III. KNEE

A. Anatomy

Imagine that you are baby-sitting a one-year-old. The baby is in a highchair and is really agitated. You decide to evaluate the baby's condition. You first evaluate if the

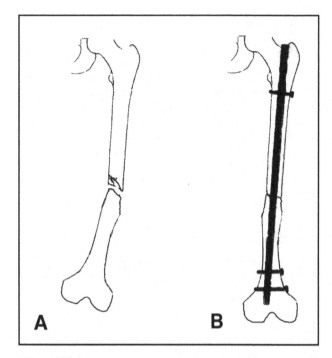

Fig. 3-7 Femoral fracture. A: Displaced mid-shaft femoral fracture. **B:** Intra-medullary nailing.

baby is sitting comfortably and if he is properly strapped in. You also evaluate the highchair itself including the cushions.

The knee is analogous to this baby-sitting situation (**Fig. 3-8**). The femoral condyles (the baby's buttocks) and proximal tibia (the seat of the highchair) compose the knee joint (**Fig. 3-9**). These two bones are securely attached to each other by the knee capsule, the cruciate ligaments and collateral ligaments (safety harness of

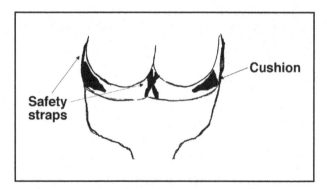

Fig. 3-8 Highchair analogy. Posterior view of a baby's bum sitting on a highchair with safety straps passing between the legs.

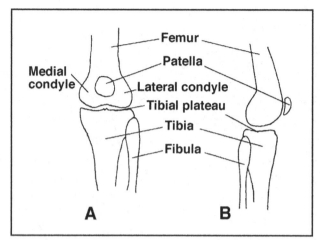

Fig. 3-9 Knee anatomy. A: Anterior view. **B:** Lateral view.

the chair). The menisci (the chair cushions) are two "C"-shaped cartilaginous spacers between the femur and tibia (**Fig. 3-10**). They act as shock absorbers. The vascular supply to the leg comes from the tibial artery, which passes directly behind the knee. Therefore, it is very susceptible to trauma. The common peroneal nerve passes laterally 2 cm below the fibular head and is also at risk for injury.

B. Approach

To distinguish among the different knee conditions, ask about the presentation of pain. Sudden and severe pain with a trauma history will suggest disruption of a ligament, meniscus, or osseous structure. Chronic symptoms will suggest a degenerative condition. The localization of the pain is also indicative since medial or lateral pain is a sign of collateral and meniscus injuries, whereas anterior knee pain relates mainly to patello-femoral conditions. Pain worse with weight bearing suggests mechanical pathologies (meniscus tear, ligament tear, or fracture). Night pain and stiffness are signs of inflammatory pathologies. Remember that hip and lumbar pathologies can cause diffuse and poorly localized knee pain.

With the patient standing:

1. Inspection: –alignment (*genu valgum, genu varum, genu recurvatum*)
   –posterior aspect for *Baker's cyst* (contained synovial fluid extravasation seldom apparent in the knee fold that is rarely symptomatic)
   –quadriceps atrophy
   –gait analysis

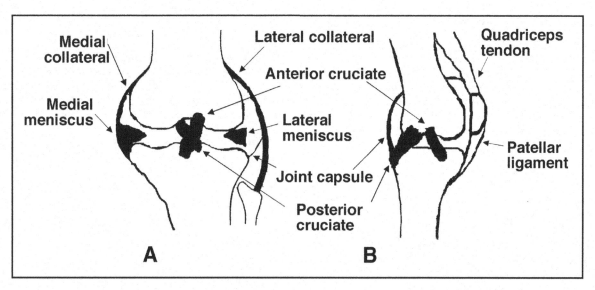

Fig. 3-10 Knee ligaments and menisci. A: AP view. **B:** Lateral view.

With the patient lying down:

1. Inspection: –skin lesion
   –muscular atrophy
   –flexum (knee cannot lie flat on the exam table)
   –swelling

2. Palpation:
   i) knee in extension: –warmth
      –effusion
      –rubbing the patella against the femur
      –behind the knee
   ii) knee in flexion: –proximal tibial edge (articular line)
      –collateral ligaments (internal/external)
      –quadriceps and patellar tendons

3. Range of motion (active/passive)

4. Specific maneuvers: –flow sign to rule out effusion (**Fig. 3-11**)
   –*Drawer test* (cf. cruciate ligament injury)
   –*Lachman test* (cf. cruciate ligament injury)
   –stress in valgus and varus (cf. collateral ligament injury)
   –*J sign test* (cf. patellar dislocation)

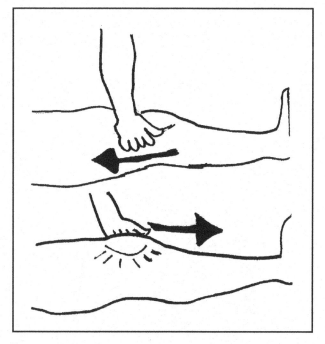

Fig. 3-11 Flow sign. The examiner rubs the medial aspect of the knee with a proximally directed motion to push the intraarticular fluid and then rubs the lateral aspect of the knee with distally directed motion to see bulging on the medial side of the knee, indicating significant knee effusion.

C. Specific Problems

1. Meniscal tear

Meniscal tears (analogous to a ripped highchair cushion) usually occur while standing up from a crouching position or from a twisting motion at the knee. The medial meniscus is more frequently torn, since it is less mobile due to its attachment with the medial collateral ligament.

Clinical Findings

The patient may present with intermittent swelling of the knee and locking. The pain is usually felt on the medial aspect of the knee. The extension of the leg may be limited due to interposition of the torn meniscus. The articular line is painful to palpation on the side of the meniscal tear.

Simple X-ray views of the knee are not revealing. MRI is the most reliable diagnostic modality.

Treatment

Conservative approach. When there is no apparent locking of knee motion, the inflammation is controlled with NSAIDs, ice and rest. Progressive weight bearing using crutches is allowed. Physical therapy helps restore full range of motion and strength.

Surgical approach. Locking of the knee is a relative emergency and must be taken care of rapidly. Persistent pain with recurrent swelling is the most frequent indication for surgery. The surgery consists of an arthroscopic repair or partial removal of the torn meniscus.

2. Ligamentous injury (Highchair lesions)

a. Cruciate ligaments

A cruciate ligament tear (broken harness between baby's legs) may occur after a twisting motion during sports activity associated with a sudden stop or hyperextension of the knee.

b. Collateral ligaments

Collateral ligament tears (broken lateral safety strap) can be isolated or associated with other injuries (**Fig. 3-12**). Medial collateral ligament tears are more frequent and occur with sudden stress on the lateral side of the knee (valgus deforming energy). A tear of the lateral collateral ligament is less common; it requires a great amount of energy hitting the inside of the knee (varus deforming energy).

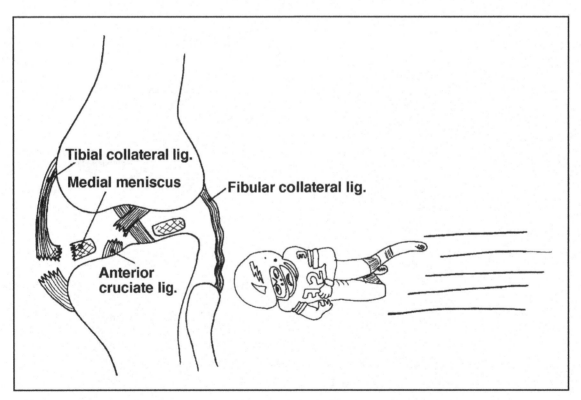

Fig. 3-12 Terrible triad of O'Donnohue. Severe lateral impact on the knee can cause a medial collateral ligament tear, meniscal tear, and ACL tear.

Clinical Findings

With ligamentous injury, and typically for the anterior cruciate ligament, the patient may recall a "popping" sensation in the knee at the time of injury. Significant knee effusion is a consistent finding.

To examine the knee, several maneuvers can be performed. Imagine that you are testing the safety straps that pass between the baby's legs. If the baby can slide forward or backward on the highchair, it means that a safety strap is broken.

This is analogous to the *drawer test,* which evaluates the cruciate ligaments by attempting to move the tibial plateau relative to the distal femur (**Fig. 3-13**). Pulling on the tibial plateau tests the integrity of the anterior cruciate ligament. Pushing on the tibial plateau tests the posterior cruciate ligament. The test is performed with the knee flexed to 90 degrees with the examiner sitting on the patient's foot. Increased tibial motion anteriorly signifies anterior cruciate injury. Increased tibial motion posteriorly signifies posterior cruciate ligament injury.

The *Lachman test* is similar but performed at 20 degrees of flexion (**Fig. 3-13**). The examiner holds the upper part of the knee in one hand and the lower part of the knee in another. With normal cruciate ligaments, a sharp end point is felt while trying to displace the proximal tibia relative to the distal femur. It is more reliable than the drawer test but difficult to do with a big leg.

Now imagine that the baby can lift her right or left buttock off the highchair by tilting sideways. It implies that a lateral safety strap must be torn. To check for a medial or lateral collateral ligament tear, stress the knee in varus and valgus to reproduce pain and assess stability.

Simple X-ray views of the knee, including oblique views are useful. An avulsion fracture at the insertion sites of the cruciate ligaments (tibial spine) may be seen. Avulsion of the lateral knee capsule is also sometimes seen (*Segond fracture*). MRI of the knee is diagnostic for cruciate ligament tears and commonly associated injuries such as meniscal and medial collateral ligament tears.

Treatment

Conservative approach. It is generally acceptable to splint the knee for 4 to 6 weeks with NSAIDs prescribed, ice and protected weight bearing with crutches. Physical therapy is started as tolerated to regain full range of motion and strengthen the surrounding muscles. Patients may desire knee bracing for sports to provide further stability and confidence.

Surgical approach. If the knee remains symptomatic and instability interferes with the practice of a sport, ligamentous reconstruction can be done using a hamstring tendon, the middle third of the patellar tendon, quadriceps tendon, or cadaver tissue (allograft). It is usually performed by arthroscopy.

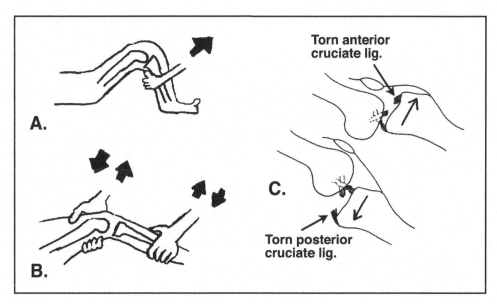

Fig. 3-13 Testing for cruciate tear. A: Drawer test performed with the knee flexed at 90 degrees. **B:** Lachman test performed while holding the knee with both hands, flexed at 20 degrees, and moving the hands in opposite direction to detect instability. **C:** Anatomic section showing tibial displacement according to the cruciate tear.

c. Knee dislocation

A knee dislocation is displacement of the tibial plateau relative to the distal femur. It implies a severe ligamentous injury and joint instability. This is analogous to a completely disrupted highchair harness with baby free to fall off the highchair.

Knee dislocation can be associated with trauma to the tibial artery (*CON lesion; c.f. Chap.1, section 3*) due to its close proximity to the bones posteriorly. **Beware!** Unrecognized vascular injury may lead to amputation!

Clinical Findings

Upon initial evaluation, the limb may be shorter. The knee is swollen and deformed. Pulses at the foot may be absent with pallor of the extremity. Common peroneal nerve injury is frequent when the tibia is dislocated posteriorly. This type of nerve injury results in a foot drop, which is the inability to dorsiflex the foot. There is also an associated loss of sensation at the base of the first and second toes.

Simple X-ray views of the knee are diagnostic.

Treatment

Conservative approach. This may be appropriate if the distal pulses are present. The dislocation should be reduced as soon as possible in the ER. Control the reduction by viewing X-rays. The limb is splinted with slight flexion at the knee. The pulses should be checked daily, since an arterial intimal tear may cause sudden occlusion of the tibial artery. The orthopedic surgeon may decide to cast the leg for 6 weeks to allow healing of the knee ligaments.

Surgical approach. If distal pulses are absent, this is a true emergency! The dislocation should be reduced immediately. The pulses may return to normal after proper realignment of the limb. If the ischemia persists, obtain an angiogram and consult a vascular surgeon, since arterial repair may be needed. The orthopedic surgeon may consider surgical stabilization by repairing the knee ligaments or stabilization with an external fixator to protect the vascular repair.

3. *Extensor mechanism injury*

a. Quadriceps rupture with patellar fracture

Quadriceps tendon and patellar tendon ruptures, together with patellar fractures or dislocation are the most frequent causes of failure of the knee extensor mechanism. Quadriceps tendon ruptures usually occur in the elderly, whereas patellar tendon ruptures usually occur in younger patients.

b. Patellar fracture

The patella (kneecap) is the largest sesamoid bone in the body. Direct trauma to the anterior knee on a dash board is a frequent mechanism. A fractured patella is by definition an intra-articular fracture and should be dealt with carefully.

c. Patellar dislocation

The usual mechanism of injury is an internal rotation of the femur with the foot fixed on the ground. This condition mainly affects teenagers.

d. Patellar tendon rupture

This injury can occur in sports when there is sudden forced flexion of the knee against a strongly activated extensor mechanism.

Clinical Findings

When the extensor mechanism is injured, complete knee extension is usually impossible or incomplete. Partial tearing of the extensor mechanism is suspected when knee extension is possible but incomplete (*extension lag*). There is usually a large intra-articular effusion.

A palpable depression is usually felt where the extensor mechanism is ruptured, such as above the patella if the quadriceps tendon is severed, between patellar fragments when the patella is fractured, or below the patella if the patellar tendon is severed. With patellar dislocation, the patella can be palpated lateral to its normal alignment with the knee. With patellar tendon rupture, the kneecap is proximally displaced (*patella alta*) from the unopposed traction by the quadriceps tendon.

Kneecap dislocation can be overlooked if the patella spontaneously reduces to its normal position. A classic sign that a dislocation has occurred is apprehension when the examiner pushes the kneecap laterally. Pain on palpation is present at the upper medial aspect of the patella since the quadriceps muscle attachment (*patellar retinaculum*) must tear to allow the patella to dislocate. Look for a positive "J sign test," which is a "J" shaped displacement of the patella as it migrates proximally and laterally upon active extension of the knee due to a weak vastus medialis or torn insertion of this muscle on the patella.

Simple X-ray views of the knee with skyline view of the patella will rule out a fractured or dislocated patella. MRI is the modality of choice to detail the location of extensor mechanism rupture. CT scan analysis can be helpful to evaluate malalignment of the patellofemoral tendon. MRI is useful for assessment of the patellar articular cartilage.

Treatment

Conservative approach. Partial tearing of the extensor mechanism with near complete extension of the leg, and a non-displaced patellar fracture can be treated with a cylinder cast for 4 to 6 weeks or with a removable splint. Physical therapy will restore strength and motion thereafter.

For patellar dislocation, the treatment consists of immobilization of the knee in 20 degrees of flexion for 3 weeks. The physical therapy can be started early, even during immobilization, to prevent quadriceps atrophy (the patient can raise the braced leg or cast while lying down).

Surgical approach. Quadriceps and patellar tendon tears with significant extension lag are treated with surgical repair of the torn tendon. The repair is protected for 4 to 6 weeks with a cylinder cast or removable splint depending on the rigidity of the repair. Physical therapy to regain full range of motion and progressive strengthening is essential.

Displaced patellar fractures (more than 3 mm displacement at the articular surface) are treated by ORIF (**Fig. 3-14**). Many techniques are possible with metallic wires, screws, or K-wires. Strong fixation allows rapid mobilization of the knee. Partial or total patellectomy is sometimes required when the fracture is highly comminuted and the fragments cannot be put back together.

Recurrent dislocation mandates surgical correction of the patella and patellar tendon misalignment. The surgery may consist of a soft tissue procedure to release the soft tissues, which are pulling the patella laterally, and tightening the soft tissue medially. A bony correction may be performed to transpose the tibial tuberosity and restore proper patellofemoral tendon alignment.

4. *Distal femoral fracture*

Clinical Findings

This injury can be associated with ligamentous injury to the knee. Definitive assessment of the ligaments can only be done after fracture reduction and stabilization.

Simple X-ray views of the knee are sufficient.

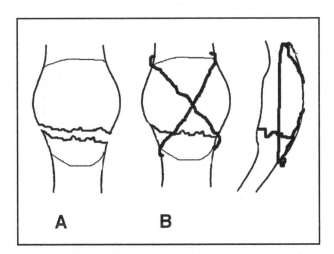

Fig. 3-14 Patella fracture. A: Displaced patella fracture. **B:** AP and lateral views of patella after ORIF with wire.

Treatment

Conservative approach. Non-displaced fractures can be treated with a cylinder cast for 6 to 8 weeks. Control X-rays are obtained weekly to pick up any displacement, which can occur inside the cast. Partial weight bearing is allowed after 3 weeks if no displacement has occurred.

Surgical approach. Intra-articular fractures with displacement of more than 3 mm at the articular surface require ORIF (**Fig. 3-15**).

5. *Tibial plateau fracture*

A tibial plateau fracture (a broken highchair) is common after a direct lateral impact at the knee level (such as a car bumper).

Clinical Findings

The common peroneal nerve is at risk for injury due to its close proximity to the fibular head. Injury to the nerve would make dorsiflexion of the foot impossible (foot drop). The ligaments of the knee are rarely torn in this case, since it is the bone that absorbs the energy.

Simple AP, lateral, and oblique views of the knee are diagnostic. A CT scan is very helpful for evaluating the degree of comminution and depression of the tibial plateau.

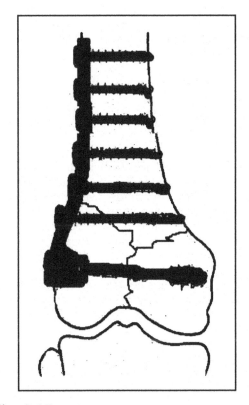

Fig. 3-15 ORIF of a distal femoral fracture.

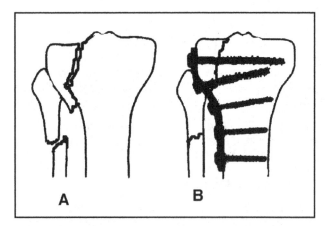

Fig. 3-16 Tibial plateau fracture. A: Displaced lateral tibial plateau fracture. **B:** ORIF.

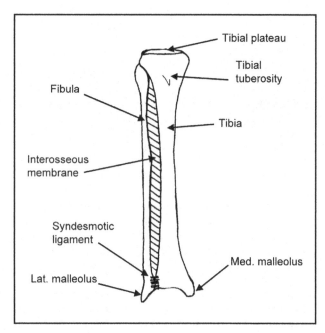

Fig. 3-17 Leg bone anatomy.

Treatment

Conservative approach. Non-displaced fractures or with a slight plateau depression of less than 3 mm can be treated with a long leg cast for 6 weeks. No weight bearing is allowed during this time to prevent any further plateau depression.

Surgical approach. Displaced fractures with more than 3 mm between the fragments are treated with ORIF (**Fig. 3-16**). Bone grafting is often necessary to fill the defect left after raising the depressed plateau. Assisted active motion is permitted when stability of the fixation is adequate. Weight bearing can be allowed 6 weeks after the fracture fixation.

IV. LEG

A. Anatomy

The leg has 2 main bones: the tibia, which supports 90% of the body weight, and the fibula on the lateral side of the leg (**Fig. 3-17**). There are 4 muscle compartments: anterior, lateral, and 2 posterior compartments. The sciatic nerve, as it descends distally behind the knee, changes its name to the tibial nerve, and provides innervation for all of the calf muscles (gastrocnemius and soleus muscles). The common peroneal nerve, which is a branch of the sciatic nerve, passes around the fibular head laterally. It provides innervation to the muscles of the lateral and anterior compartments for eversion and dorsiflexion of the foot, respectively. Injury to this nerve can cause a foot drop.

B. Approach

Assess muscles attached to the tibia and fibula, and bony integrity of the lower leg. A systematic examination with inspection, palpation, and range of motion of

the joints above and below the injury is performed. Assess neurovascular integrity of the limb.

The leg is the most common area for a compartment syndrome to occur. The clinician should remain alert for the 5 P's (Pain, Paresthesia, Palpation of a hard compartment, Paralysis, Pallor/pulselessness) of a compartment syndrome that can appear at any time after leg injury.

C. Specific Problems

1. Tibial and fibular fractures

Clinical Findings

Open fractures (*CON lesion; c.f. Chap. 1, section 3*) are common with tibial fractures. The skin over the tibia can easily be broken by the spiky tip of a fracture fragment. Traumas due to high-velocity accidents are at risk for a compartment syndrome. The 5 P's (Pain, Paresthesia, Palpation, Paralysis, Pulselessness) of a compartment syndrome must be ruled out (*CON lesion; c.f. Chap. 1, section 3*).

Simple X-ray views are sufficient for the diagnosis.

Treatment

Conservative approach. Non-displaced closed fractures are treated with a full leg cast for 6 weeks. The cast is then changed to a below knee walking cast for another 6 weeks. Follow-up X-rays are obtained weekly for

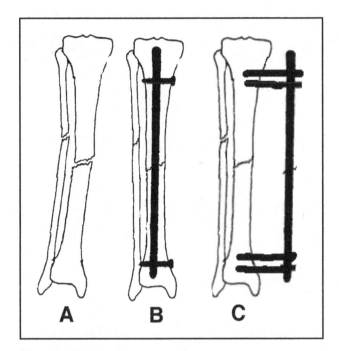

Fig. 3-18 Tibial fracture. A: Displaced tibial fracture. **B:** ORIF with intra-medullary nailing. **C:** Stabilization with an external fixator in the context of an open fracture.

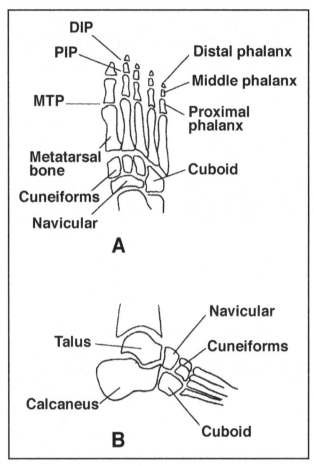

Fig. 3-19 Foot anatomy.

the first 3 weeks of treatment to confirm stable alignment. Physical therapy can be started as soon as the full leg cast is shortened to a below knee cast in order to restore muscle strength to the quadriceps.

Surgical approach. Displaced and comminuted fractures require ORIF. The most frequently used option is intra-medullary nailing (**Fig. 3-18**). Fixation of the fracture with a plate and screws is also an option but requires periosteal stripping, which causes bone devascularization and leads to a higher risk of infection and non-union. Physical therapy can be started immediately post-operatively with partial weight bearing for 6 to 8 weeks.

V. FOOT AND ANKLE

A. Anatomy

The foot is a complex structural arch, which is constantly under great loads and strains (**Fig. 3-19**). The neuro-vascular bundle passes behind the medial malleolus and supplies the plantar area. The dorsum of the foot carries the dorsalis pedis artery coming from the anterior compartment of the leg. The talar dome is squeezed between the malleoli and is almost entirely covered with cartilage. The blood supply to the talus is very precarious, especially at the neck.

The ankle joint is made of 3 bones: the tibia, the fibula, and the talus (**Fig. 3-20**). The distal tibia forms the posterior and medial malleoli. The distal fibula forms the lateral malleolus. All the bones forming the ankle joint

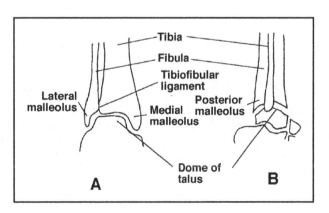

Fig. 3-20 Ankle anatomy. A: Anterior view. **B:** Lateral view.

are held together by several ligaments (**Fig. 3-21**) and form a ringlike structure (**Fig. 3-22**). The tibia and fibula are tightly bound together by the *interosseous membrane*. This membrane is thicker at the ankle and forms the syndesmotic ligaments.

B. Approach

Focus on the precise site of pain, meaning forefoot (most likely rheumatoid arthritis) or hindfoot (most likely sero-negative arthritis). Midfoot (tarsal area) pain is often due to diabetic arthropathy or stress fracture. Plantar pain is related to inflamed plantar fascia. Inspection of the patient's shoeware is also relevant.

With the patient standing:

1. Inspection: –gait analysis with bare feet for limping, flat feet, and also asking the patient to walk on tiptoes and then on heels to assess mechanical and neurological functions.

With the patient lying down:

1. Inspection: –skin lesion
   –swelling
   –deformity

2. Palpation: –warmth
   –periarticular structures (tendons, ligaments)

3. Range of motion: flexion, extension, eversion, inversion

4. Specific maneuvers:
   i) Drawer test (pulling the foot forward and backward relative to the tibia to detect instability)
   ii) Stress in valgus and varus (forcing the foot in valgus and varus position to detect instability due to incompetent ligaments)

C. Specific Problems

1. Metatarsalgia

This condition involves the area padding the metatarsal heads of the plantar surface of the foot.

Clinical Findings

Collapsing of the foot's transverse arch (degenerative flat foot) can cause pain at the level of the metatarsal heads.

Simple X-ray views of the foot will usually reveal associated hallux valgus and degenerative changes.

Treatment

Conservative approach. This approach consists of decreasing the plantar pressure on the metatarsal heads

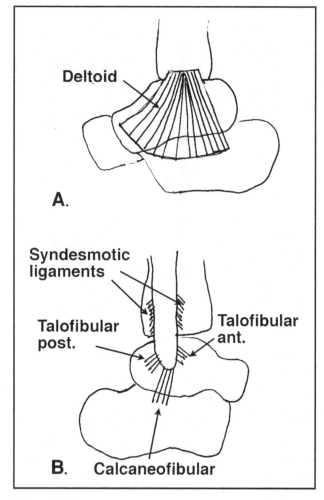

Fig. 3-21 Ankle ligaments. A: Medial view. **B:** Lateral view.

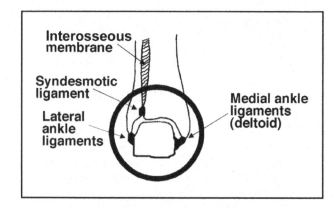

Fig. 3-22 Ankle ringlike structure. Ankle AP view showing ligaments (black thick lines) and interosseous membrane (hatched lines). The ligaments are structurally analogous to a ringlike structure.

with a plantar orthosis (metatarsal pad). The metatarsal pad is placed in the shoe and supports the plantar arch and the metatarsals, but leaves the metatarsal heads free hanging.

Surgical approach. Surgery is mainly considered for rheumatoid arthritis or poliomyelitis patients. It consists of doing metatarsal osteotomies to relieve the pressure on the metatarsal heads.

2. *Hallux valgus*

This condition is common in older women. It has a strong familial trait.

Clinical Findings

There is a lateral deviation deformity of the first toe with bony prominence of the first metatarso-phalangeal joint known as a *bunion* (**Fig. 3-23**). There is severe pain over the bunion. Shoe wear often becomes problematic.

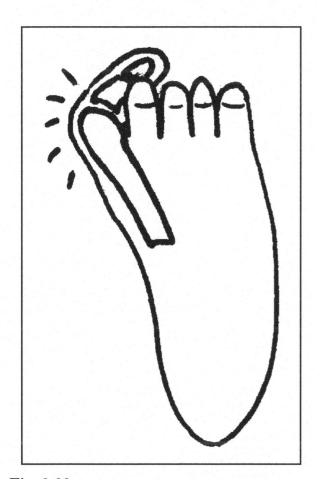

Fig. 3-23 Bunion. The hypertrophied metatarsal head of the first toe creates a deformation known as a bunion.

Treatment

Conservative approach. Orthopedic shoes with a large toe box can be helpful. The idea is to relieve pressure on the 1st metatarso-phalangeal joint to alleviate inflammation.

Surgical approach. Patients with painful deformities can undergo soft tissue surgery with or without osteotomy of the first metatarsal bone to normalize alignment. Resection of the metatarso-phalangeal joint (resection arthroplasty) is reserved for elderly patients who are often more inactive. Surgical correction for cosmesis is not advised since the toe may become painful after surgery.

3. *Heel pain and plantar fasciitis*

Plantar fasciitis is an inflammation of the plantar fascia at its insertion on the calcaneum (**Fig. 3-24**).

Clinical Findings

The pain is present when standing and decreases when no weight is applied on the plantar surface of the foot. It is reproducible on palpation over the heel pad. A flattened plantar arch may cause great tension on the plantar fascia and ultimately bring heel pain.

Simple X-ray views of the foot may show a calcaneal spur, which has not been proven to be of clinical significance.

Treatment

Conservative approach. New shoes with good arch support may suffice. Added arch support insoles are also a good alternative. Gel heel pads are also available.

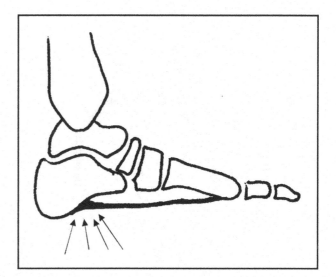

Fig. 3-24 Plantar fasciitis. Stress at the point of insertion of the plantar fascia on the calcaneum (multiple black arrows) causes painful inflammation.

Resolution of pain may take up to a year. Local steroid infiltrations are generally not routine due to reported fat pad necrosis.

Surgical approach. Persistent pain lasting more than a year can be surgically treated with plantar fascia release from the calcaneal spur.

4. Ankle sprain and fracture

Trauma can disrupt the ringlike structure of the ankle either through the ligaments, bones, or both (**Fig. 3-25**). When the ring is partially disrupted, the ankle remains stable. When the ring is totally disrupted, the ankle joint is likely to be unstable.

Clinical Findings

Use the *Ottawa ankle rule* (sounds like "ought to walk") to clinically differentiate between an ankle sprain and a fracture. Ask the patient to walk. If the patient can walk at least 4 steps on the injured foot, the ankle is not broken and the patient does not need X-rays. If the patient cannot walk, an X-ray is needed to exclude a fracture. Patients with fractures also tend to have pain at the posterior aspect of the injured malleolus whereas ligamentous injuries tend to give more anterior pain, especially directly over the torn or partially torn ligaments: tibio-talar, calcaneo-peroneal, and tibio-fibular.

Pain on palpation over the proximo-lateral aspect of the leg may signify an associated proximal fibular fracture.

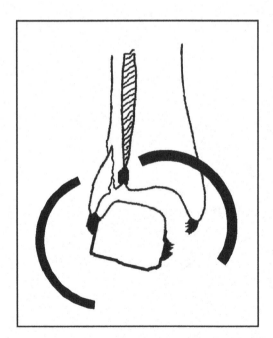

Fig. 3-25 Ankle fracture. An ankle fracture is analogous to a broken lifesaver, which usually breaks at 2 places.

With a twisting injury, the energy can tear the syndesmotic ligaments, travel up the leg to disrupt the interosseous membrane, exit close to the knee, and cause a fracture of the proximal fibula (*de Maisonneuve's fracture*).

Simple X-ray views of the ankle with an added view of the ankle joint space (mortise) in slight internal rotation (mortise view) are used to assess for fractures. An asymmetrical mortise signifies ankle instability. The lateral view will help assess for the integrity of the posterior lip (posterior malleolus). If the fibula is fractured 2 cm or more above the mortise, then suspect an injury to the syndesmotic ligaments. When a de Maisonneuve fracture is suspected, an X-ray of the leg will show a fracture of the proximal fibula.

Treatment

Conservative approach. A mild ankle sprain can be treated with progressive weight bearing as tolerated. More severe cases require splinting or a cast with a rubber heel (walking cast) to control pain, and to provide stability for the ligaments to heal. Non-displaced fractures are treated with a non-walking cast for 6 weeks. Follow-up X-rays the following week are necessary to rule out displacement of the fracture. The cast might be loose due to decreasing swelling and may need to be changed. After 4 to 6 weeks of immobilization, the cast is removed and a control X-ray should be taken to assess fracture healing. Physical therapy is often necessary to restore strength, motion, and sense of position (proprioception).

Surgical approach. Displaced fractures with an asymmetrical mortise view require ORIF. The ankle is then splinted until the control visit the following week. An X-ray will ascertain stable alignment. The sutures are then removed and a non-walking cast is applied to complete 6 weeks of immobilization. Some surgeons may feel confident about their ORIF and allow immediate gentle motion of the ankle.

When the syndesmotic ligaments are torn, a screw is added just above the mortise to reapproximate the tibia and fibula, allowing the ligaments to heal (**Fig. 3-26**). This screw is often removed 2 to 3 months post-op since it is at risk of breaking due to the normal micro-motion between the tibia and fibula.

5. Talus fracture

This type of fracture is often seen when pressing the brake pedal on a car trying to avoid an accident. The impact can cause a forceful dorsiflexion of the foot and ultimately fracture the talus.

Clinical Findings

The blood supply to the talus is precarious, and therefore, avascular necrosis (AVN) of the talus is a frequent post-traumatic complication.

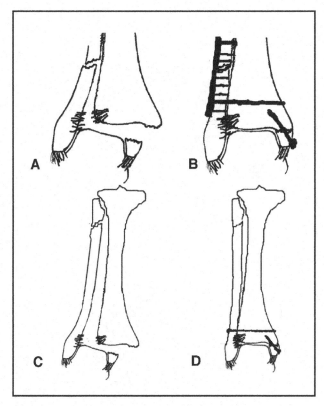

Fig. 3-26 Syndesmotic ligaments rupture. A: Displaced ankle fracture with syndesmotic ligaments rupture. **B:** ORIF with syndesmotic screw. **C:** De Maisonneuve's fracture. **D:** ORIF with syndesmotic screw around the ankle.

Simple X-ray views of the foot and ankle joints including a mortise view are diagnostic. The fracture line is typically found at the talar neck. A CT scan will reveal the fracture pattern for pre-operative planning.

Treatment

Conservative approach. Non-displaced fractures are treated with a non-walking cast for 6 weeks. One week post injury, a follow-up X-ray should be done to rule out displacement. The cast must be changed if it loosens, since swelling is expected to decrease.

Surgical approach. Displaced fractures are treated with ORIF (**Fig. 3-27**). Anatomic repositioning will reduce the risk of AVN of the talus.

6. Calcaneal (lover's) fracture

This injury typically occurs after a fall from a height much like a lover jumping over a balcony in order to avoid an encounter with a furious husband.

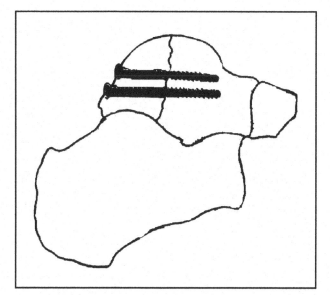

Fig. 3-27 ORIF of a talus fracture.

Clinical Findings

The injury is often bilateral and the swelling is often very impressive. Associated injuries are typically ankle fractures and thoraco-lumbar burst fractures (see Axial skeleton Chapter 4). Therefore, pain on palpation over the thoraco-lumbar area is due to a fractured vertebra until proven otherwise and must be considered as a potential risk for spinal cord injury (*CON lesion; c.f. Chap.1, section 3*).

Simple X-ray views including an oblique image of the foot and dedicated heel views are required. On the lateral view, assessment of the Bohler angle will evaluate the extent of displacement (**Fig. 3-28**). Simple spine

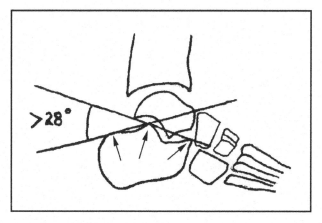

Fig. 3-28 Bohler angle. Normal Bohler angle of 28 degrees. This angle is traced using the 3 bony prominences (black arrows) of the calcaneum. A smaller angle signifies a flattened calcaneum (displaced fracture).

views over the painful area are obtained for screening. A CT scan will provide details about the structural integrity of the involved vertebra.

Treatment

Conservative approach. The primary line of treatment is to wrap the foot with soft roll and elastic bandages. The foot is elevated to decrease the swelling. Weight bearing is rarely possible before 8 to 12 weeks. Early mobilization will prevent stiffness.

Surgical approach. Severe displacement with flattening and widening of the calcaneus can prevent normal shoe wear. ORIF will restore the calcaneal architecture (**Fig. 3-29**).

7. *Lisfranc fracture*

A *Lisfranc fracture* is, in fact, a fracture/dislocation between the tarsal and metatarsal bones (**Fig. 3-30**). This injury is rare, but can occur with a fall on the foot while it is pointing down. It can also occur from forceful pressing on a car brake pedal. Jacques Lisfranc de St. Martin (1790-1847), a French army surgeon, used to do amputations through this joint on the battle field (*Lisfranc amputation*).

Clinical Findings

The swelling may be mild, but there is intense pain while applying torsion maneuvers to the forefoot. Pain out of proportion to the apparent injury may signal a compartment syndrome (*CON lesion; c.f. Chap.1, section 3*) of the foot and warrants immediate orthopedic consultation.

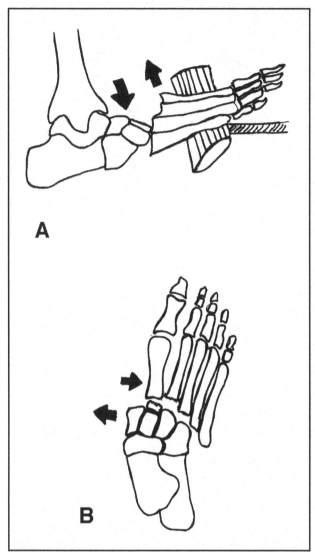

Fig. 3-30 Lisfranc fracture-dislocation. A: Brake pedal injury with dorsal displacement of the forefoot. **B:** Lateral displacement of the forefoot with fracture of the base of the second metatarsal.

Simple X-ray views with oblique images of the foot will help make the diagnosis. A fractured base of the second metatarsal is often associated with a Lisfranc fracture. When the X-ray is equivocal, MRI can be obtained for ligamentous assessment.

Treatment

Conservative approach. A Lisfranc injury requires non-weight bearing casting for 6 to 8 weeks. Prolonged residual pain is possible.

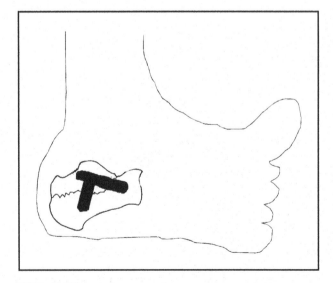

Fig. 3-29 ORIF of a calcaneal fracture.

Surgical approach. Surgical treatment is recommended for displaced ligamentous lesions of the forefoot. The surgery consists of screw fixation to stabilize the mid-tarsal bones (**Fig. 3-31**).

8. *Fifth metatarsal base fracture (Jones' fracture)*

A Jones' fracture is a stress fracture of the fifth metatarsal base. It is more common in athletes.

Clinical Findings

The ecchymosis may be quite impressive.
Simple X-ray views of the foot are diagnostic.

Treatment

Conservative approach. Fifth metatarsal fractures are rarely displaced enough to require surgical attention. A walking cast for 4 to 6 weeks may or may not decrease pain associated with walking. A light splint for one or two weeks, with progressive weight bearing using crutches is also a safe method and decreases the significant risk of deep vein thrombosis.

Surgical approach. Severe displacement of the fifth metatarsal base or painful non-union may require ORIF. A walking cast for 4 to 6 weeks or crutches without weight bearing will provide safe ambulation after surgery.

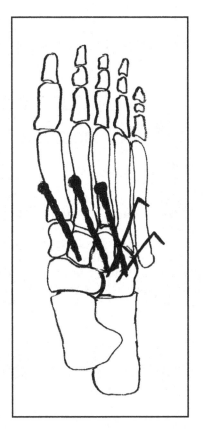

Fig. 3-31 **ORIF of a Lisfranc fracture-dislocation.** ORIF with screws and K-wires.

CHAPTER 4. AXIAL SKELETON

I. SPINAL COLUMN

A. Anatomy

Cervical spine

Imagine a Greek statue representing the Titan "Atlas," who is supporting the earth's weight as a punishment from Zeus (**Fig. 4-1**). The Titan is sitting on a stool on top of a Greek column. The work is made of 7 marble blocks. The top one is sculpted into Atlas. The block under Atlas includes a stool, which serves as a supporting axis for the statue. Atlas's massive feet rest on the edges

of this second block (**Fig. 4-2**). All other blocks are cemented one on top of each other to make a column.

The cervical spine is structured in much the same way as the above Greek statue. Seven cervical vertebrae, numbered 1 to 7 from top to bottom, are stacked on top of each other to make a column (**Fig. 4-3**). Notice the cervical column is slightly curved posteriorly. The top vertebra is called "Atlas" (C1) after the famous Titan. It sits on "Axis" (C2), which has a stool-like protrusion, called the *odontoid process*. Much like the Titan's massive feet, Atlas's lateral masses rest on the edges of Axis. In addition, this column is held in place by several ligaments and cementlike spacers (the intervertebral disks), which separate each vertebra.

Thoraco-lumbar spine

The thoraco-lumbar spine is composed of 12 thoracic vertebrae (T1 to T12 from top to bottom) and 5 lumbar vertebrae (L1 to L5 from top to bottom) (**Fig. 4-4**). Each vertebra is separated by intervertebral disks much like the

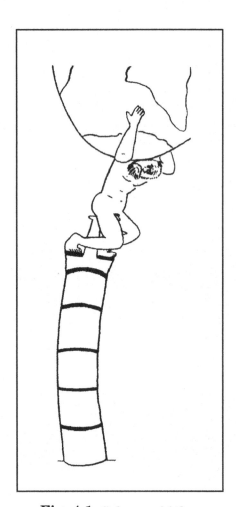

Fig. 4-1 Column of Atlas.

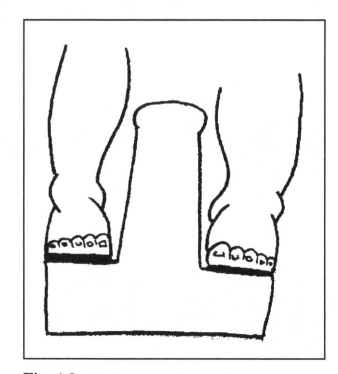

Fig. 4-2 Atlas's massive feet analogy.

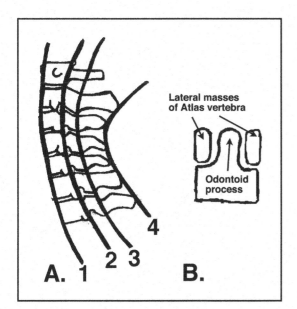

Fig. 4-3 Cervical spine. A: Alignment of the 7 cervical vertebrae. *Line 1*—alignment of the anterior vertebral body wall. *Line 2*—alignment of posterior vertebral body wall. *Line 3*—spinolaminar line. *Line 4*—spinous process line. **B:** Cross section of the Atlas and Axis vertebrae.

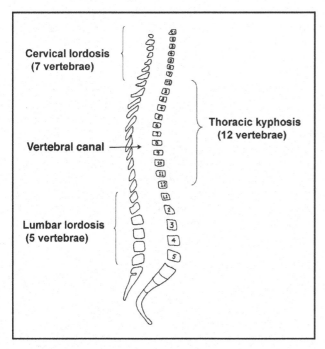

Fig. 4-4 Complete vertebral column. Cross section of the vertebral column showing the vertebral bodies, vertebral canal and spinous processes.

cervical spine. The thoracic spine is concave anteriorly (*kyphosis*) and the lumbar spine is concave posteriorly (*lordosis*). The intervertebral disk has a central core called the *nucleus pulposus*, which is surrounded by a ring of collagen named the *annulus fibrosus*. Mechanically, the vertebral column has 3 pillars consisting of the vertebral bodies, the pedicles, and laminae (**Fig. 4-5**). The spine is considered unstable when there is an injury to 2 or more pillars.

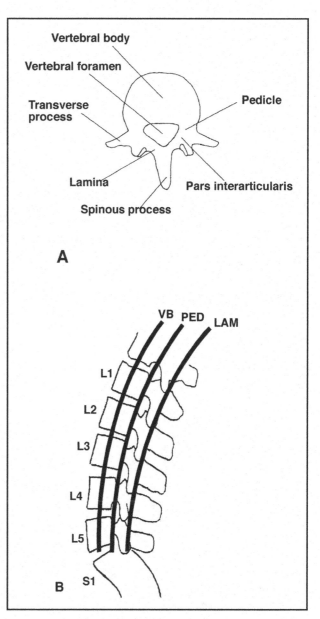

Fig. 4-5 Vertebral body alignment. A: Typical vertebral body. **B:** Lateral view of vertebral bodies with illustration of the 3 pillars (thick black lines: *VB*—vertebral bodies, *PED*—pedicles, *LAM*—laminae) as main mechanical support structures.

Spinal cord

Imagine a power bar that supplies electrical current to a computer and all its peripheral devices. This is analogous to the spinal cord supplying current to the limbs (**Fig. 4-6**). In the vertebral canal runs the spinal cord from which exit the spinal nerve roots. Two nerve roots exit to either side of the spinal cord at each vertebral level. At the cervical level, there are 8 nerve roots for 7 vertebrae, so that each nerve root exits above its respective vertebra, except for the 8th nerve root, which exits under the 7th cervical vertebra (**Fig. 4-7**). Therefore all the subsequent nerve roots of the spinal cord exit below their respective vertebra. The termination of the spinal cord is called the *conus,* which is typically located at L1/L2. At the conus, multiple nerve roots emerge (*cauda equina*). Knowledge of the dermatome and main muscle groups is essential (**Fig. 4-8**).

B. Approach

The site of maximal pain helps identify the cause of cervical pain (*cervicalgia*). Ask about headaches and ear pain, which can be referred from higher levels of cervical nerve irritation (C1, C2, C3, C4). Lower cervical pain with irradiation to the arm or upper back may originate from the lower cervical vertebrae (C5, C6, C7, C8). Ask about paresthesia, limp muscles, and sphincter weakness.

For lower back pain (*lumbalgia*), the age of onset and the duration are important to investigate. Lumbar pain with onset in the early twenties and lasting beyond 3 to

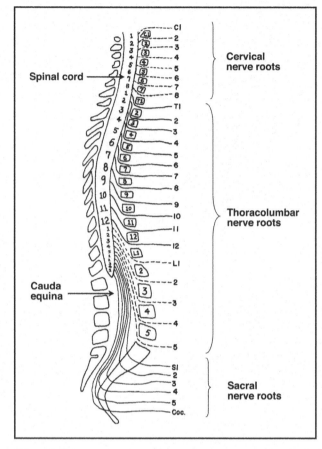

Fig. 4-7 Spinal cord. Spinal cord with exiting nerve roots and corresponding vertebra.

6 months is indicative of inflammatory conditions, whereas mechanical pathologies can occur at all ages and are shorter lasting, with pain during the day that worsens with physical exertion. Pain generated from compression of the spinal cord or nerve roots may be exacerbated by coughing, defecation, or Valsalva maneuver. Lower limb paresthesia, anesthesia of the perineum, or sphincter malfunction are indicative of significant compression of the neurological elements. Rapid deterioration of the symptoms represents a medical emergency (*CON lesion; c.f. Chap.1, section 3*).

In Non-traumatic Circumstances

With the patient standing:

1. Inspection: —position of the head and lordosis of the neck
   —for kyphosis, scoliosis, hypo/hyper lumbar lordosis
   —muscular spasms
   —gait analysis

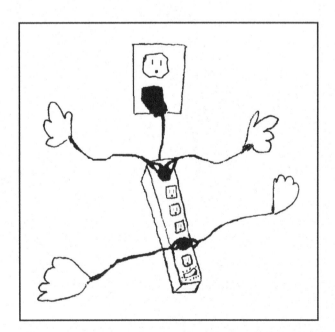

Fig. 4-6 Power bar analogous to the spinal cord.

ROOT	SENSORY	MOTOR	REFLEX
C3-4-5	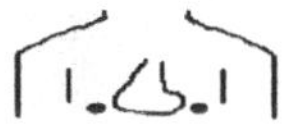	Diaphragm excursion	
C4	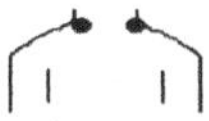	Shrug shoulders	
C5	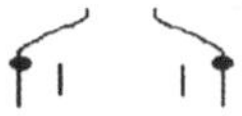	Deltoid contraction	Biceps
C6	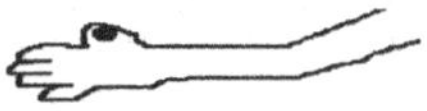	Elbow/Wrist flexion	Forearm
C7	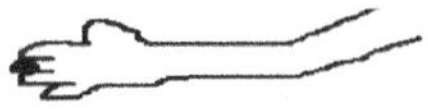	Elbow/Wrist extension	Triceps
C8	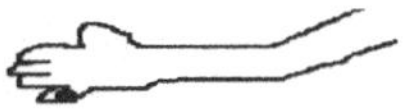	Finger abduction	
L1	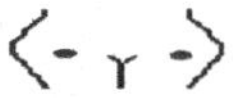	Hip flexion	
L3	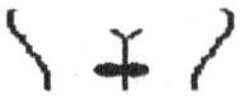	Knee extension	Patellar tendon
L4	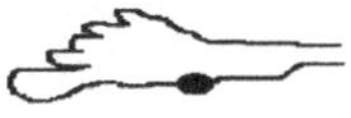	Ankle dorsiflexion	Patellar tendon
L5	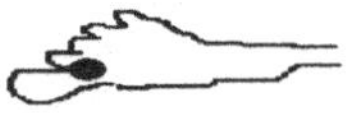	Big toe extension	
S1	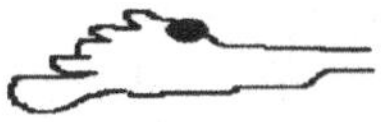	Ankle plantarflexion	Achilles tendon (ankle jerk)
S2-3	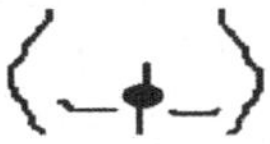	Anal sphincter	Bulbo-cavernous

Fig. 4-8 Nerve root normal function.

2. Palpation: –spinous processes

3. Range of motion (active/ passive): flexion, extension, lateral bending, rotation

4. Specific maneuvers: –*Schober test* (**Fig. 4-9**)

With the patient lying down on stomach over a pillow when no history of trauma:

1. Inspection: –skin lesion
   –swelling
   –deformation

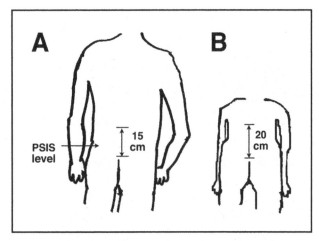

Fig. 4-9 Schober test. The Schober test is performed to assess the lumbar spine range of motion. **A:** The patient stands erect with normal posture. Identify level of posterosuperior iliac spine (PSIS). Mark midline at 5 cm below iliac spine. Mark midline at 10 cm above iliac spine. **B:** Patient bends at waist to full forward flexion. Measure distance between 2 lines (started 15 cm apart). The normal distance between 2 lines should increase to >20 cm. When the distance does not increase to >20 cm, it suggests decreased lumbar spine range of motion.

2. Palpation: –warmth
                –spinous processes
                –para-spinal muscles
                –sacro-iliac joints

3. Range of motion (active / passive) of the hips: flexion, extension, rotation

4. Specific maneuvers:
   i) *Lasègue maneuver*
   ii) *tripod maneuver* (**Fig. 4-10**)
   iii) complete neurological exam (motor, sensory, reflexes)

In Trauma Circumstances

The approach is similar with the exception that the patient is usually strapped to a safety board when first seen in the emergency room. The inspection of the neck and back must be performed with mobilization of the patient as a unit with the help of many orderlies. After visual inspection and palpation, the patient is returned in a supine position to complete the physical examination.

Imagine a short circuit in the power bar such that there is no current to supply the peripherals of your computer. This is analogous to a complete spinal cord injury, which implies a complete loss of motor function or sensitivity distal to the lesion. An incomplete spinal

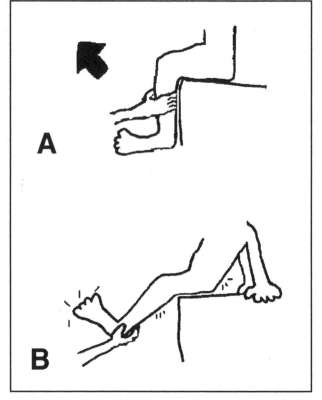

Fig. 4-10 Tripod maneuver. A: With the patient sitting at the edge of the exam table, lift the leg upward to trigger or reproduce sciatalgia. **B:** When the symptoms appear, the patient will throw himself backward, with the hands acting as a tripod to alleviate the pain shooting down the leg.

cord lesion implies that there is preservation of some movement and sensitivity distal to the lesion (e.g., toe movement, anal sphincter contraction and sensation). Spinal cord injuries are frequently seen after motor vehicle accidents (MVA), diving or falling from a height. Therefore, when a spinal cord injury is suspected, the clinician must check each nerve root territory for abnormal function with regard to:

1. Skin sensitivity
2. Muscle contraction
3. Tendon reflexes

The skin sensitivity can be tested by touching softly or pricking gently with a needle in the corresponding dermatome for each nerve root.

Any muscle weakness is graded according to the following scale:

Grade 0: no contraction
Grade 1: trace of contraction

Grade 2: movement with gravity eliminated
Grade 3: movement against gravity
Grade 4: movement against resistance
Grade 5: normal strength.

Tendon reflexes are evaluated for symmetry and intensity by gentle tapping with a reflex hammer.

Testing the *bulbocavernous reflex* will help determine the presence of a "SPINAL SHOCK", which can occur after a trauma to the spinal cord. A spinal shock can mimic a complete spinal cord injury (areflexia, flaccidity, and hypotension) and may last up to 24 hours.

The bulbocavernous reflex is evaluated by compressing the tip of the penis or gently pulling on the foley catheter and feeling for a contraction of the anal sphincter. If this reflex is absent during the first 24 hours after a spinal injury, the overall neurological status and exam may not be reliable. No definitive prognosis can be made because the spinal cord is in spinal shock. When the bulbocavernous reflex is present, it means that the spinal shock is over. If there is no neurological recovery by then, the prognosis is poor.

Spinal cord injuries (*CON lesion; c.f. Chap.1, section 3*) warrant immediate consultation with an orthopedic surgeon or neurosurgeon, since delay in treatment may worsen the prognosis for recovery.

Treatment

Conservative approach. Part of the conservative approach to spinal cord injury consists of giving high doses of steroids with the hope of diminishing the inflammatory response and injury to the spinal cord. Treatment length and timing remain controversial.

Surgical approach. The surgical approach consists of removing any compressing structure from the spinal cord as soon as possible. The spinal column must then be stabilized to prevent any further injury to the spinal cord. In some cases, removal of a vertebral body (corpectomy) may be necessary. Instrumentation with rods, pedicular screws, and bone grafting are used to restore stability.

C. Specific Problems

1. Vertebral disk disease

A herniated disk can occur at any level of the spine, but is most frequent at the lumbar level following a strenuous effort or after a torsion motion.

Clinical Findings

The patient may complain of an acute back pain, but pain radiating to the leg (sciatica) is the main finding. Pain usually radiates distal to the knee on the posterolateral side of the leg and possibly up to the toes. Val-salva maneuvers (sneezing, coughing, and constipation) may reproduce the symptoms. Posture changes such as loss of lordosis and scoliosis are often due to muscular spasms. Muscle weakness and paresthesia can be observed along a precise nerve root.

The reflexes are asymmetric and weak (hyporeflexia) on the affected side. The *tripod maneuver* is positive (see **Fig. 4-10**), meaning that the patient leans back on his upper limbs while in a sitting position when one leg is extended. The *Lasègue maneuver*, which is performed by lifting the patient's leg while supine, will reproduce the radiating pain.

Fecal incontinence, urinary retention, and loss of perianal sensitivity are classic symptoms of a disk hernia at the level of the conus (*CON lesion; c.f. Chap.1, section 3*). This means that the herniated disk is squeezing the tip of the spinal cord. Damage at this level may be irreversible and requires urgent decompression. The *cauda equina syndrome* occurs when the hernia is located slightly distally to the conus. Symptoms are similar to compression of the conus, but are usually reversible.

Simple X-ray views of the thoraco-lumbar spine can reveal disk space narrowing at the affected level. MRI and CT are diagnostic for disk hernia and nerve root compression.

Treatment

Conservative approach. For a cervical hernia, a soft cervical collar will reduce movements of the cervical spine and provide comfort. NSAIDs, mild narcotics, physiotherapy, and massage therapy are also helpful.

A painful lumbar disk hernia with mild neurological deficit is treated with analgesia, NSAIDs, and epidural steroid injection to decrease inflammation around the nerve root. The bulging disk may shrink with time, and the symptoms may disappear.

Surgical approach. Surgery is considered when there are severe symptoms: mainly pain and weakness in one or both limbs. It consists of removing the diseased disk by an anterior approach through the neck for a cervical hernia and through a posterior approach for the lumbar hernia. When there is compression of the spinal cord, conus, or cauda equina, urgent surgery is indicated.

2. Spondylolysis/listhesis

Spondylolysis is a defect in the pars interarticularis and usually occurs at L5 (**Fig. 4-11**). When a spondylolysis is present, the affected vertebral body is only held against the rest of the vertebra by ligaments and the intervertebral disk. With time, this superior vertebral body slips forward on the inferior one. This process is called *spondylolisthesis* (**Fig. 4-12**). These injuries mostly appear after extreme repetitive movements of the spine such as in gymnastics.

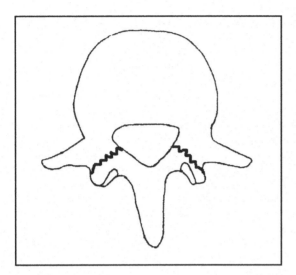

Fig. 4-11 Pars interarticularis defect. Vertebral body with fractured pars interarticularis bilaterally (thick black zigzag).

Clinical Findings

With spondylolysis, pain is usually localized to the lower lumbar area and is aggravated with lumbar extension. There are usually no neurological symptoms.

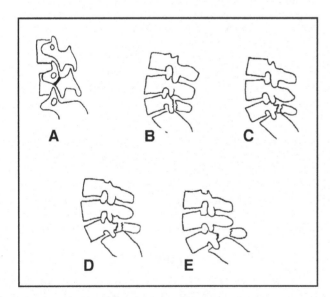

Fig. 4-12 Spondylolysis and spondylolisthesis.
A: Appearance of a collar on the neck of the scotty dog on the oblique lumbar view is diagnostic of spondylolysis. **B:** Grade 1 (<25% slippage). **C:** Grade 2 (>25%, <50% slippage). **D:** Grade 3 (>50%, <75%). **E:** Grade 4 (>75% slippage).

When spondylolisthesis occurs, neurological symptoms usually signify an advanced degree of slippage.

Simple X-ray views of the lumbar spine, including oblique views, are required. In equivocal cases, a CT scan may be obtained.

Treatment

Conservative approach. The main treatment is analgesia and modification of activities.

Surgical approach. Surgery is considered for young individuals with uncontrollable symptoms. Stabilization of the affected spinal segment is done with bone grafting only or with bone graft and instrumentation. Surgery can prevent further slippage of the spondylolisthesis. Reduction of the spondylolisthesis is not recommended.

3. Spinal stenosis

Spinal stenosis is a narrowing of the spinal canal and usually occurs in elderly patients.

Clinical Findings

Typically, patients have insidious and progressive lower back pain. Pain can radiate to one or both legs. Lower limb cramps usually occur after walking one or two blocks (*claudication*). Sitting down or bending forward can bring symptomatic relief by increasing the spinal canal diameter. This relieves pressure on the spinal nerves (the cauda equina). The neurological exam is usually normal at rest, but a partial deficit may be noticeable after a walk.

The tripod and Lasègue maneuvers are generally negative.

Simple X-ray views of the lumbar spine including oblique views are obtained. Osteophytes, disk space narrowing, sclerosis of vertebral end plates, and hypertrophy of articular facets are usually present. CT scan of the lumbar area will reveal stenosis of the spinal canal (diameter < 8 mm). MRI of the lumbar area is ideal to show intervertebral disk disease and compression of the cauda equina.

Treatment

Conservative approach. This approach includes NSAIDs, rest, steroid injection of the facets, physiotherapy and walking aids.

Surgical approach. When neurological findings or claudication is significant, the alternative approach consists of decompression of the central canal by partial or total removal of the lamina at the level of the stenosis (*laminectomy*). Instrumentation with rods, pedicular screws and bone grafting may be used to improve spinal stability.

5. Cervical fracture and dislocation

Clinical Findings

You are Jefferson, a famous architect working with a sculptor called Cervico Spinous. Your task is to determine if the Greek column you are restoring is stable or not. When you first arrive on site, you have no idea whether the column is stable. The first thing to do is to put a supporting scaffold in place to avoid further damage (**Fig. 4-13**). This is analogous to putting a cervical collar on the patient to provide proper protection (**Fig. 4-14**). You are now ready to start your assessment.

On gross inspection, if the Earth supported by Atlas the Titan is in an abnormal position, there may be instability of the Greek column. Similarly, patients with an abnormal head position may have a fracture or dislocation of the cervical spine. The neurological exam detailed in the previous section (cf. spinal cord injury) will help evaluate the presence of associated neurological lesions.

You then proceed to meticulous inspection of the Greek column to rule out the presence of cracks in the marble blocks and signs of instability. This is analogous to obtaining plain X-rays of the cervical spine in order to look for unstable fractures and dislocations.

Simple X-ray views of the cervical spine include a lateral, frontal, and open-mouth view. The entire cervical spine should be visible on the X-ray. Cervical X-ray is an important radiological exam to learn. Refer to *Clinical Radiology Made Ridiculously Simple* for a basic ap-

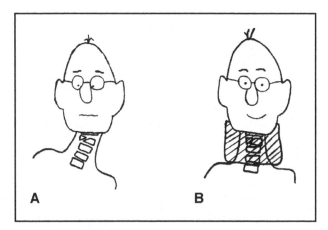

Fig. 4-14 Cervical splinting. A: Cervical fracture unprotected. **B:** Cervical fracture protection with collar.

proach to this exam. Any suspected fracture is further evaluated with a CT scan.

Unstable Cervical Fractures (Fig. 4-15)

a. Flexion tear drop fracture

A *flexion tear drop fracture* is secondary to a flexion injury. It is extremely unstable and severe, and therefore should not be confused with the more benign extension tear drop fracture. It results in disruption of all ligaments as well as the intervertebral disk at the level of injury. A small fragment of the antero-inferior portion is broken off of a vertebral body with posterior displacement of the vertebral body itself. This type of fracture often results in anterior spinal cord compression.

b. Hangman's fracture

A *hangman's fracture* is secondary to an extension injury, which commonly occurs in MVAs or in hangings (hence the name). It is a bilateral C2 pars interarticularis or pedicle fracture, with anterior displacement of the anterior part of C2.

c. Hyperextension fracture-dislocation

A *hyperextension fracture-dislocation* is secondary to an extension injury and is unstable. It results in a slight anterior vertebral subluxation, with a complex fracture near the articular surfaces.

d. Burst fracture

A *burst fracture* results from an axial injury (just like a Jefferson's fracture). It causes a compression of the vertebral body and results in loss of both anterior and posterior vertebral body height. This is unlike the wedge fracture, in which there is only loss of anterior vertebral

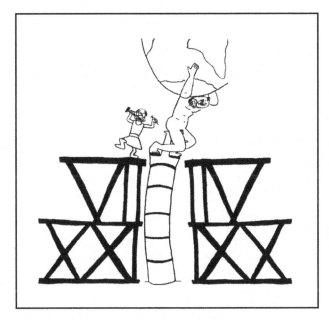

Fig. 4-13 Column of Atlas with supportive scaffold.

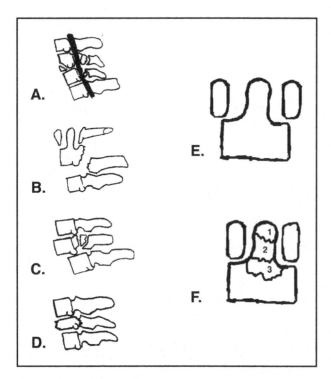

Fig. 4-15 Unstable cervical fractures. A: Flexion tear drop (spinal cord as a thick black line). **B:** Hangman's. **C:** Hyperextension fracture-dislocation. **D:** Burst. **E:** AP view of a Jefferson's fracture. **F:** AP view of odontoid fractures (1-mid-odontoid, 2-base, 3-through body of axis).

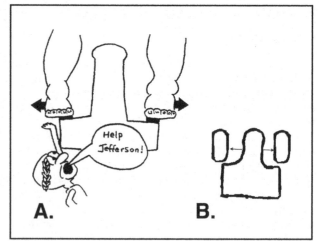

Fig. 4-16 Jefferson's fracture analogy. A: Atlas's massive feet are slipping of the column and the sculptor Cervicos Spinos is asking Jefferson the architect for the help. **B:** Open-mouth view of a Jefferson's fracture with displacement (black arrow) of the lateral masses of Atlas vertebra relative to the Axis vertebra.

body height. Bony fragments may push on the spinal cord and cause symptoms. This type of fracture is most commonly located in the mid-cervical spine. It is also associated with calcaneal fractures, which results from a fall from a great height (see Lower Limb chapter).

e. Jefferson's fracture

Jefferson's fracture is analogous to Atlas's massive feet slipping off the edges of the second block (**Fig. 4-16**). Look at the open-mouth view to see if the Atlas's lateral masses have slipped sideways and therefore are no longer flush with the Axis edges. This unstable fracture is secondary to an axial injury. Examples of axial injuries include having a heavy object fall on one's head or diving into a shallow pool. It consists of at least two fractures of C1. A rigid ring structure cannot be broken in only one spot. Try breaking a lifesaver in only one spot—it's impossible!

f. Odontoid fracture

An *odontoid fracture* is analogous to a crack in the Titan's stool. Look at the open-mouth view for a black line

in the odontoid process, which represents a fracture. This unstable fracture is secondary to a multidirectional injury and is a fracture of the odontoid process of C2. There are three types of odontoid fractures. Type 2 is the most unstable of the odontoid fractures.

Stable Cervical Fractures (Fig. 4-17)

a. Clay shoveler's fracture

This stable fracture is secondary to a flexion injury. It involves an avulsion of a piece of the spinous process and most frequently occurs in the lower C-spine. It is best seen on the lateral view.

b. Wedge fracture

This stable fracture is the result of a flexion injury. It involves compression of the anterior part of the vertebral body and therefore is best seen on the lateral view.

c. Extension tear drop fracture

This stable fracture is the result of an extension injury. It is an avulsion of a piece of the antero-inferior portion of a vertebra and often occurs at C2.

Dislocations

a. Atlanto-occipital dislocation

Atlanto-occipital dislocation is analogous to the Titan Atlas, dropping the Earth. It is a dislocation at the junc-

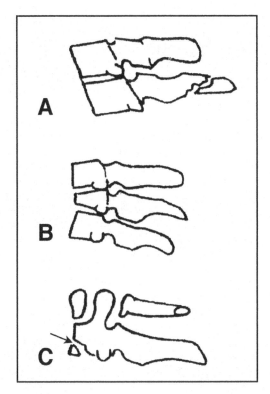

Fig. 4-17 Stable cervical fractures. A: Clay shoveler's. **B:** Wedge. **C:** Extension tear drop (black arrow).

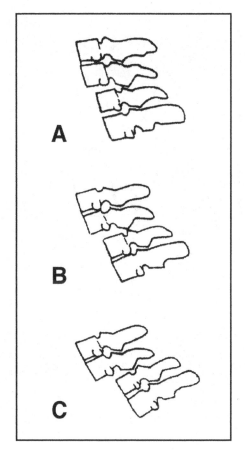

Fig. 4-18 Facets dislocations. A: Subluxed facets. **B:** Perched facets. **C:** Locked facets.

tion between the Atlas vertebra and the skull. This injury often results in death. The anterior dislocation is much more frequent and much easier to see on x-ray. It usually gives rise to an increase in prevertebral soft tissue swelling.

b. Facet joint dislocations (**Fig. 4-18**)

Facet dislocation is analogous to misaligned blocks in our Greek column. It is best seen on the lateral view as a step deformity within the vertebral alignment. A step deformity of >3 mm is always abnormal and means that the spine is likely unstable. Facet dislocation occurs secondarily to hyperflexion of the cervical spine. This hyperflexion results in disruption of the anterior longitudinal ligament, intervertebral disk, and posterior ligaments.

There are 3 types of bilateral facet dislocations, all of which are unstable. They are, in order of increasing severity: the *subluxed facets, the perched facets, and locked facets.*

Treatment

Conservative approach. Stable non-displaced fractures can be treated with rigid cervical collar for 6 to 8 weeks. A halovest (**Fig. 4-19**) is mainly considered for non-displaced odontoid fractures.

Surgical approach. Unstable or displaced fractures are treated with ORIF. The removal of the vertebral fragments (*corpectomy*) will decompress the spinal cord and allow for potential recovery.

6. Thoraco-lumbar fracture

In the emergency room, the patient must remain supine at all times and can only be mobilized as a unit with help from orderlies for clinical assessment.

Clinical Findings

The paramedic's spinal board must be removed as soon as possible to prevent pressure sores. While removing the board with the orderlies, one might take the opportunity to inspect the back for deformation and bruises.

Localized pain on palpation of a spinal segment is always suspicious for fracture. Vertebral spinous process malalignment or increased space between processes is also suggestive, as are ecchymoses and hematoma. The

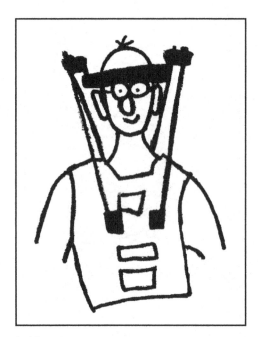

Fig. 4-19 Halo vest. Screws secure a ring structure (halo) to the head, and metal rods secure the halo to a vest around the chest to stabilize the cervical fracture.

neurological exam detailed in the previous section (cf. spinal cord trauma) will help evaluate the presence of associated neurological lesions.

Order simple X-ray views of the thoraco-lumbar spine and views centered over the suspected fractured vertebra. A CT scan will further document the injury and assess stability.

On the frontal view of the spine, each vertebra looks like an owl (**Fig. 4-20**). Each eye represents a pedicle, and the beak of the owl represents the spinous process. When an X-ray of the spine is taken obliquely, each vertebra takes on the appearance of a Scottie dog (**Fig. 4-20C**). Each part of the dog corresponds to a component of the vertebra. Therefore, the Scottie dogs are standing on each other's ears and tails to form the intervertebral articulation. The body of the Scottie dog corresponds to one of the laminae, the eye is one of the pedicles, the nose is one of the transverse processes, and the neck is the pars interarticularis. The ears and the tail are the superior intervertebral articular processes; the front legs and hind legs represent the inferior intervertebral articular processes (**Fig. 4-21**). If the behind of the Scottie dog is located to the right, you are looking at the right lamina, pars interarticularis, and pedicle, and vice versa.

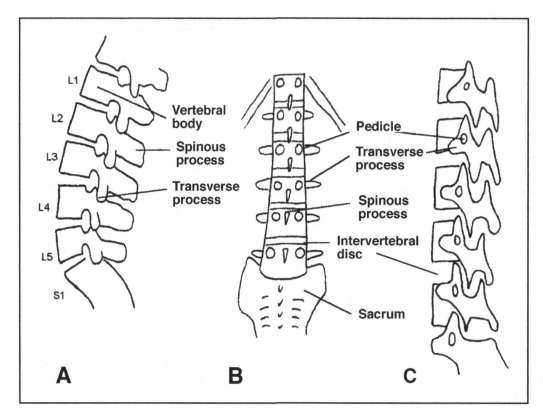

Fig. 4-20 Thora-columbar spine. A: Lateral view. **B:** AP view. **C:** Oblique view.

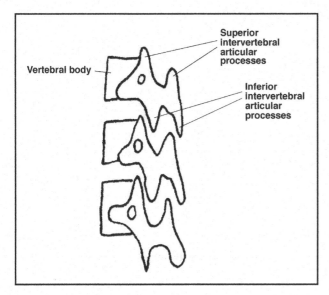

Fig. 4-21 Scottie dog. Close-up of an oblique view of the lumbar spine.

Unstable Thoraco-Lumbar Fractures

a. Chance fracture

A *Chance fracture* results in the horizontal severing of a vertebra (**Fig. 4-22**). Ligaments are disrupted, and the fracture line may even go through the intervertebral disk. Chance fractures are best seen on a lateral view of the spine. Sometimes when the fracture line extends through the spinous process, one can see the two distinct pieces on the frontal view. It looks like there are two spinous processes at one level (as if the beak of the owl at the af-

fected level is open). This unstable injury is often the result of an MVA, when a lap belt immobilizes the pelvis, while the rest of the upper body is thrust forward.

b. Burst fracture (Don Juan fracture)

A *burst fracture* results in the collapse of an entire vertebral body (**Fig. 4-23**). On a lateral view, the heights of the anterior and posterior wall of the vertebral body are smaller in comparison to adjacent normal vertebrae. Fragments extending into the spinal canal are common and may cause neurological damage. On the frontal view, the interpedicular distance may be increased. The mechanism of injury is a fall from a height (a jump from a balcony).

Stable Thoraco-Lumbar Fractures

a. Wedge fracture

A *wedge fracture* results in the collapse of the anterior vertebral body. On the lateral view, there is decreased height of the anterior wall of the vertebral body in comparison to the adjacent normal vertebrae. The posterior wall of the vertebral body is intact. The spinal canal is not involved, and there is no neurological damage. A wedge fracture is a hyperflexion injury.

b. Spinous process fracture

In this injury, there is a black fracture line in the spinous process. The spinal canal and the stability of the spine are unaffected.

Treatment

Conservative approach. Stable fractures are immobilized with a brace called the *Thoraco-Lumbar Spinal*

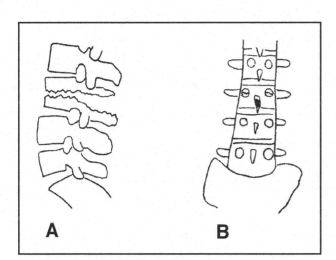

Fig. 4-22 Chance fracture. A: Lateral view. **B:** AP view.

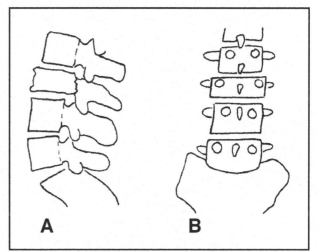

Fig. 4-23 Burst fracture of L3. A: Lateral view. **B:** AP view.

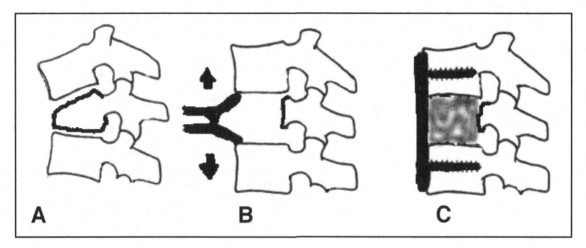

Fig. 4-24 Burst fracture management. A: Cord compression due to vertebral collapse. **B:** Corpectomy and decompression. **C:** Bone grafting and ORIF.

Orthosis (TLSO) for 8 to 12 weeks. The patients are encouraged to walk as tolerated, and physical therapy is started when the orthosis is removed.

Surgical approach. Unstable fractures are treated with ORIF (**Fig. 4-24**). When neurological symptoms are present, decompression of the neural structures by removing the broken vertebral body (corpectomy) is necessary. The surgeon may decide to stabilize the spine with metal rods, pedicular screws and bone graft.

II. PELVIS

A. Anatomy

The pelvis basically looks like a big "pretzel." It is composed of three rings, which make one central pelvic inlet, and two obturator canals (**Fig. 4-25**). Directly beneath

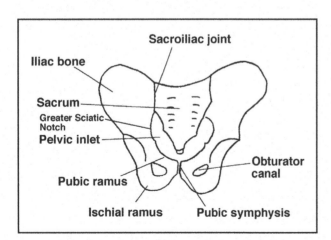

Fig. 4-25 Pelvic anatomy.

the fifth lumbar vertebra is the sacrum, which is composed of 5 fused vertebrae and the coccyx. The sacrum is bordered on each side by the iliac wings, which creates the pelvic inlet. The iliac wings are contiguous with the acetabulum, which contains the femoral heads, and the ischio-pubic rami. All the muscles providing motion to the hip are attached to the pelvis. The sciatic nerve exits the pelvis through the greater sciatic notch. The femoral nerve and artery enter the anterior aspect of the leg by passing under the inguinal ligament.

B. Approach

The Unstable Patient

In a trauma patient with persistent hypotension, the traumatologist or orthopedic surgeon must eliminate pelvic fracture as a source of bleeding. If the pelvis seems unstable upon palpation, it can be temporarily held together with a piece of fabric tied around the hip while waiting for the trauma X-ray series (cervical spine, chest, and pelvis). The orthopedic surgeon will apply an external fixator to stabilize the fracture and ultimately contain the bleeding of the pelvic vessels.

The Stable Patient

After stabilization of the vital signs, the physical exam is performed in a systematic manner.

1. Inspection: –skin lesion
   –swelling
   –deformity, leg length inequality

2. Palpation: –warmth
   –periarticular structures (tendons, ligaments, sacroiliac joints, pubis)

66

3. Range of motion of the hips: flexion, extension, eversion, inversion

4. Specific maneuvers: –pressure applied to the iliac wings to detect instability

C. Specific Problems

1. Pelvic ring fractures

"Don't break the pretzel!"

The pelvis is a strong and rigid structure and requires tremendous force to be disrupted. Fractures mainly occur in car accidents. Injury to the pelvis can be life threatening because there may be extensive hemorrhage.

Clinical Findings

Signs of pelvic injury are unequal leg length, pain on palpation of the iliac crests, limping, or inability to walk. The neurovascular status of the lower limbs must be as-sessed. Fracture edges may injure adjacent structures. For example, blood at the urinary meatus or coming from the Foley catheter may imply a ruptured bladder. Blood on vaginal or rectal exams may also imply injuries to these structures.

Simple X-ray views of the pelvis should include AP, oblique (*Judet*) views, and inlet and outlet views of the pelvis. When a pretzel breaks, it usually breaks at 2 places due to its rigidity. The pelvic ring behaves in a similar manner. Always look for a second fracture line on the X-ray.

A CT scan is extremely valuable for detailed analysis of a fracture seen on simple films. It helps to determine the residual stability of the pelvis.

Unstable Pelvic Fractures (Fig. 4-26)

a. Malgaigne fracture

A *Malgaigne fracture* involves fractures through an ischiopubic ramus (or the pubic symphysis) and the

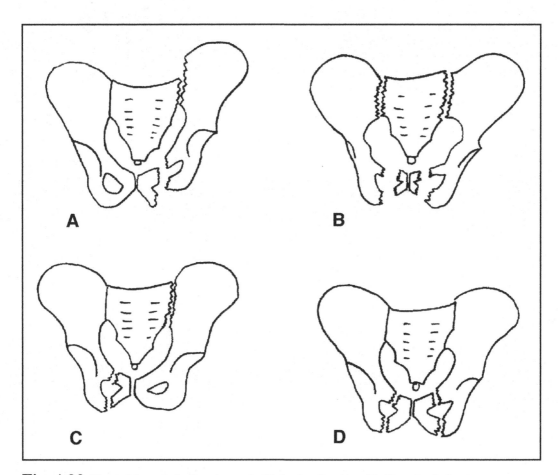

Fig. 4-26 Unstable pelvic fracture. A: Malgaine fracture. **B:** Open book fracture. **C:** Bucket handle fracture. **D:** Straddle fracture.

sacroiliac joint on the same side. Fracture fragments can be displaced vertically.

b. Open book fracture

An *open book fracture* refers to fractures through the ischiopubic rami (or pubic symphysis) and SI joints on both sides. The pelvis is cracked open like a book.

c. Bucket handle fracture

A *bucket handle fracture* involves fractures through the ischiopubic rami on one side and a SI joint fracture on the opposite side.

d. Straddle fracture

A *straddle fracture* goes through both ischial rami and pubic rami. The small piece of bone containing the pubic symphysis is free to move.

Stable Pelvic Fractures

a. Ramus fracture

Ramus fractures can be located on both the ischial ramus and pubic ramus, and are stable. Ramus fractures in young individuals are usually due to MVA and are associated with serious complications. This injury is relatively frequent in the elderly population due to osteoporotic bone. The pain is reproduced by direct palpation on the ischium. It is very difficult to get these patients out of bed to walk due to pain. Hip motion is usually tolerable. Pain is not precisely localized to the groin area as it is for a hip fracture.

b. Avulsion fracture

An *avulsion fracture* occurs when a small chip of bone is pulled off at the origin or insertion site of a tendon.

Simple X-ray views of the pelvis are diagnostic.

Treatment

Conservative approach. Non-displaced fractures of the iliac wing and stable fractures of the pelvic ring can be treated with narcotics, NSAIDS, and rest. Progressive mobilization with crutches or a walker is introduced as the pain becomes tolerable.

Surgical approach. Unstable pelvic ring fractures and displaced acetabular fractures must be surgically treated for optimal results. The surgery consists of application of an external fixator, or ORIF with plates and screws (**Fig. 4-27**).

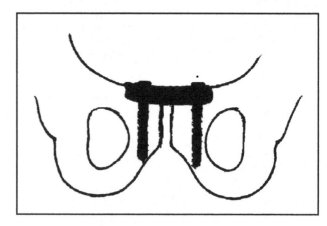

Fig. 4-27 Symphysis pubis ORIF. Stabilization of the symphysis pubis with plate and screws. Severe displacement may require additional plate and screws.

CHAPTER 5. SYSTEMIC CONDITIONS

I. INFECTION

1. Septic Arthritis

A *septic arthritis* means infection within a joint. Bacteria may enter a joint space through a puncture wound or through the blood (hematogenous seeding). The enzymes generated from the bacteria or by the immune response fighting the infection may permanently damage the cartilage and destroy the joint (**Fig. 5-1**). Septic arthritis is therefore considered an emergency. It can occur in any joint of the body.

Clinical Findings

The involved joint is warm and erythematous. There is extreme tenderness on palpation and the patient won't let you move the joint. The fever is sustained, with elevated neutrophils on blood work.

Definitive diagnosis is made with joint aspiration, gram stain, and culture of the sample. When the sample is on its way to the lab, empirical antibiotics are started (e.g., cefazolin 1 gram IV q8h). After looking at the gram stain and cultures, the microbiologist will determine the proper antibiotics for the definitive therapeutic regimen.

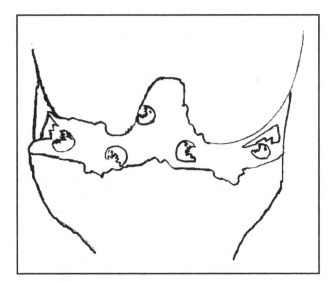

Fig. 5-1 Septic arthritis. Bacteria inside a joint, such as the knee, can chew up the cartilage and menisci.

X-rays of the involved joint can reveal intra-articular effusion, joint space narrowing, and eventually, articular destruction.

Treatment

Conservative approach. A conservative approach is not standard. Repeated joint aspirations and IV antibiotics may be considered.

Surgical approach. The joint is opened (*arthrotomy*) to allow aggressive lavage with several liters of water. A drain is left in place for subsequent effusion to drain spontaneously. Lavage in the OR may be repeated as needed.

2. Osteomyelitis

Osteomyelitis implies infection in the bone. As with septic arthritis, bacteria may enter the bone from a direct puncture injury or through hematogenous seeding. Ends of long bones in children are particularly vulnerable to hematogenous seeding, due to sluggish blood flow as blood circulation makes a U-turn when reaching the growth plate (**Fig. 5-2**). Osteomyelitis can cause formation of necrotic bone (*sequestrum*) (**Fig. 5-3**). As pus accumulates under pressure, it can erode bone and create an abcess under the periosteum. The abscess can also burst into the joint if the capsule is nearby to complicate the condition with septic arthritis.

Clinical Findings

As pus increases pressure inside the bone, the pain becomes more severe. Fever and chills may be present. There is usually swelling, redness, and warmth superficially over the infected bone. Limping or inability to use the involved body part is frequent. If pus is oozing from skin (*sinus tract*), gram stain and cultures are ordered. An empirical antibiotic, such as cefazolin, is started after the cultures are obtained and sent to the lab. After looking at the gram stain and cultures, the microbiologist will determine the proper antibiotics for the definitive therapeutic regiment.

X-rays of the involved area are required to rule out the presence of bone destruction (*osteolysis*) or a sequestrum (necrotic bone bathing in pus). A CT scan will better define the infected area and also allow for a

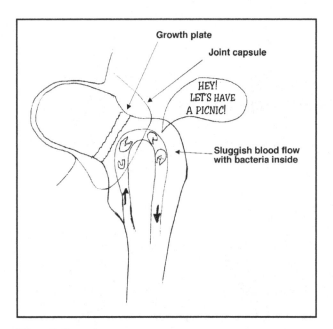

Fig. 5-2 Dramatization of blood flow to pediatric hip. The slow blood flow at ends of long bones due to U-turn blood circulation may predispose bacterial seeding at the metaphyseal level of the proximal femur of children.

biopsy. MRI can evaluate the infection in bone and adjacent soft tissues, but the edema and inflammation may result in overestimation of the extent of the infection. In the first 7 to 10 days, a bone scan with gallium can pinpoint the location of a subclinical infection not yet apparent on X-ray.

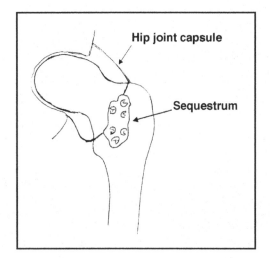

Fig. 5-3 Osteomyelitis. Infection at the metaphysis of the proximal femur.

Treatment

Conservative approach. This approach can be considered when no bony osteolysis is visible on X-ray. A trial of 6 weeks of antibiotics can be successful. A negative bone scan and non-progressive bony erosion on X-rays will prove the efficacy of the therapy.

Surgical approach. Surgery is considered as soon as bony erosion is visible on X-rays. Open debridement and irrigation is done. Several debridement attempts may be required. Amputation up to normal viable tissue level is sometimes performed. At least 6 weeks of IV antibiotics is administered to surgical patients.

II. ARTHRITIS

There are several types of arthritis, all of which ultimately lead to the destruction of the joint.

1. Osteoarthritis

Osteoarthritis (OA) is wear and tear or degenerative disease of the cartilage. It mainly occurs with old age, overuse, or as a consequence of a trauma to the articular cartilage (intra-articular fracture). The cartilage can be affected by the liberation of proteolytic enzymes, released by the chondrocytes, destroying the collagen and proteoglycans. Therefore, OA is primarily a cartilage disease with a secondary synovitis. OA is not considered a systemic disease.

Clinical Findings

The pain is usually mechanical, as overuse will trigger inflammation of the involved joint. Advanced destruction of the joint by arthritis ultimately causes pain even at rest. The swelling (intra-articular effusion) and limitation of range of motion are also proportional to the severity of the disease.

X-rays of the involved area may reveal thinning of the joint space, periarticular osteophytes, sclerosis of the joint line, and periarticular cystic lesions.

Treatment

Conservative approach. The initial treatment consists of avoiding overuse of the involved joint, and if needed, complete rest. NSAIDs and steroid injections are extremely helpful.

Surgical approach. Joint replacement (*arthroplasty*) is the most successful technique (**Fig. 5-4**). It is the most common orthopedic procedure nowadays with great results, which are pain relief and near normal joint function. The complication rate is low with less than 1% infection rate as the norm. Joint fusion (*arthrodesis*) will prevent movement between the worn-out surfaces and also stop the pain.

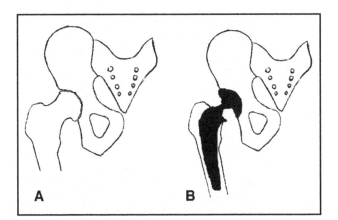

Fig. 5-4 OA of the hip. A: Arthritic hip with absent joint line and marginal osteophytes. **B:** Total hip prosthesis composed of a hemispheric acetabular component and femoral stem.

2. Rheumatoid arthritis (RA)

Rheumatoid arthritis (RA) is an autoimmune disease involving overproduction of antibodies, which target the synovial lining of joints and tendon sheaths. The inflammatory tissues (*pannus*) secondarily affect bone and cartilage. It can be a slow, indolent process or extremely aggressive and disabling.

Clinical Findings

Hand involvement classically affects the wrist, MP, and PIP joints. The fingers can ultimately deviate towards the ulnar side of the hand (*ulnar drift*). *Boutonnière* (**Fig. 5-5**) and *swan neck* (**Fig. 5-6**) deformities of

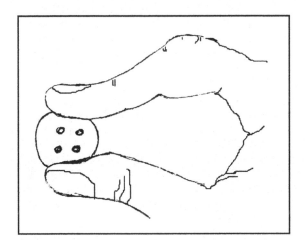

Fig. 5-5 Boutonnière deformity. Holding a button between the index finger and the thumb simulates the fixed finger found in patients with rheumatoid arthritis.

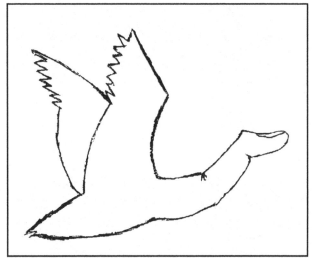

Fig. 5-6 Swan neck deformity. A swan neck simulates the fixed finger deformity found in patients with rheumatoid arthritis.

the fingers are due to ligament disruption around the IP joints. Extensor tendon rupture of the fourth and fifth fingers may occur due to tendon erosion over the inflamed distal radio-ulnar joint at the wrist level.

The cervical spine is mostly affected at the atlanto-axial joint. This joint has a small synovial membrane that can become inflamed and damaged at the transverse ligament, which holds the odontoid to the Atlas cervical vertebra. Parasthesia, paralysis, or sudden death can occur secondary to cervical spinal cord compression due to dislocation of vertebral bodies.

RA is a systemic disease with extra-articular manifestations such as fatigue, weight loss, and subcutaneous nodules.

X-rays are diagnostic. There are periarticular erosions, marked osteopenia, and ultimately severe destruction of the joint architecture. Cervical spine views are mandatory before any surgical intervention requiring an intubation.

Complementary exams include lab work that may reveal anemia of chronic disease, presence of rheumatoid factors, elevated sedimentation rate.

Treatment

Conservative approach. The goal of conservative treatment is to suppress the immune system to avoid any further joint destruction. NSAIDs, steroid infiltrations, immunosuppression with systemic steroids, gold salts, and anti-malarial agents are all immunosuppressive drugs with differing potency. Splinting of the affected limb can provide structural support and pain relief. Consultation with a rheumatologist will provide proper follow-up.

Surgical approach. When the drugs are no longer effective or when a joint is severely damaged, the only remaining option is surgery. It mainly consists of removal of the hypertrophied synovial lining (*synovectomy*) in the affected joint or tendon sheath, replacement of the joint surfaces with a prosthesis (**Fig. 5-7**), or fusion of the joint (*arthrodesis*). Joint replacement for arthritic hips and knees is a routine orthopedic procedure with great pain relief and near normal joint function restoration. Infection rate after joint replacement is about 1%.

3. Crystal arthropathy (Gout, Pseudo-gout, Hydroxyapatite crystal disease)

Of all the crystal arthropathies, gout is the only one characterized with a constant anomaly in serum analysis, which is a high level of uric acid, although only 10 to 15% of people with hyperurecemia will develop an articular pathology. The majority of gout cases can be explained by renal hypoexcretion. The concentration of uric acid plasma is determined by a balance between absorption, production, destruction, and renal excretion. Uric acid is the final product of purine metabolism.

Crystal arthropathies have in common that they present themselves in an acute episode under the form of a mono-arthritis (the big toe for gout) or poly-arthritis, of short duration but recurrent. Evolution to a chronic presentation with crystal deposits is the exception (10 to 25% of the clinical cases). At puberty the circulating levels of uric acid are set in males and at menopause for females. High plasma uric acid levels can be asymptomatic for 20 years before the first crisis, which explains symptoms appearing at 35 to 40 years old in males and 65 to 70 in females. Hyperuricemia is often linked with other medical problems, such as hypertension, coronary heart disease, obesity, diabetes, and hyperlipemia.

Clinical Findings

Signs and symptoms of crystal arthropathies can be similar to septic arthritis with swelling, warmth, and redness of the joint, and possible low-grade fever.(cf. Chapter 5, Septic arthritis).

During an acute crisis of gout, there is phagocytosis of crystals and secretion of inflammatory mediators. At physiologic pH, uric acid is in the urate form. If the concentration increases, the coefficient of solubility is surpassed and urate precipitates to form crystals. The crystals are phagocytosed and lysosomal enzymes and chemotactic factors are liberated, attracting more polymorphonuclear cells.

Simple X-ray during an acute crisis is often normal. In chronic or recurrent cases, there is articular bony erosion and soft tissue deposits (*tophi*) classically affecting the first metatarso-phalangeal joint (big toe).

Complementary exams will reveal an elevated serum uric acid level. A 24 hour urine collection will diagnose abnormal uric acid excretion. Analysis of the synovial fluid of the affected joint will determine the pathology. Under the microscope, gout crystals are yellow and birefringent under the polarized light of the microscope. A neutrophil that phagocytosed an oversized needle-shaped urate crystal is a common sight.

Pseudo-gout (calcium pyrophosphate dihydrate-CPPD) can appear in the same condition as gout, but mainly affects the knees. It appears on simple X-rays as calcified and fibrous cartilage (chondrocalcinosis). There are no blood serum levels that are diagnostic. Hydroxyapatite crystal disease is a crystal arthropathy that can occur suddenly. Women aged between 30 and 45 are mostly affected. It usually causes a monoarthropathy with classic signs of inflammation (calor, rubor, pain). The hydroxyapatite deposits can be found in or around the joints, such as tendons and ligaments.

Treatment

Conservative approach. A gout crisis can be ended with colchicine, which will block the leukocyte action of adherence, migration, lysosomal granule movement on the cytoskeleton, and liberation of chemotactic factors. Allopurinol is a drug that inhibits the enzyme xanthine oxidase, which transforms hypoxanthine and xanthine into uric acid.

Pseudo-gout and hydroxyapatite crystal disease respond well to NSAIDs.

Surgical approach. Surgery is rarely needed. It may be required to relieve the pain from a destroyed joint by doing a resection of the affected joint (*resection arthroplasty*), fusion (*arthrodesis*), or joint replacement (*arthroplasty*).

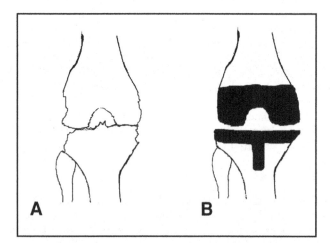

Fig. 5-7 RA of the knee. A: Destruction of the joint architecture and periarticular erosions. **B:** Total knee prosthesis with femoral component, polyethylene spacer (not visible on X-ray) and tibial component.

III. METABOLIC BONE DISEASE

Bone is a metabolically active tissue. Throughout life bone is laid down by osteoblasts and dissolved by osteoclasts. Cancellous bone, which is the soft matrix of bone, is metabolically more active than cortical bone (bone hard white shell) and therefore more prone to anomalies when metabolic disorders occur. Many factors can affect bone homeostasis.

1. Osteoporosis

In osteoporosis, the bone that is present is normal but insufficient in quantity, and therefore at increased risk of breaking. Osteoporosis occurs mainly in menopausal women and the elderly (*senile osteoporosis*), and is due to an imbalance between bone resorption and bone deposition. In women, peak bone mass is 20% less than in men at maturity. There is an accelerated bone loss at menopause (up to 1% loss per year), which mainly affects cancellous bone. Senile osteoporosis affects both cancellous and cortical bone. Both types can surely coexist. Risk factors for osteoporosis are numerous (**Fig. 5-8**).

Clinical Findings

Osteoporosis is insidious and asymptomatic until a trivial fall occurs, such as tripping on the edge of the car-pet. The most frequent presentation is a broken femoral neck (see Hip fracture, Lower Limb chapter) or a distal radius fracture (see Colles' fracture, Upper limb chapter). Other typical injuries are vertebral column fractures and pelvic ischium fractures.

Simple X-rays of the area of concern are ordered. CT scanning may be indicated. In advanced cases, the bone appears relatively dark on the X-rays because of low bone density (*osteopenia*). The diagnostic test of choice is a bone density scan. This exam is performed with a specialized instrument that calculates the bone density at the hip and lumbar spine level. A curve with percentiles relative to normal bone is generated. Critically low bone density levels are associated with higher fracture rates.

Laboratory tests are usually normal.

Treatment

Conservative approach. The approach to osteoporosis is mainly conservative. The non-pharmaceutical regimen is a balanced diet rich in calcium and regular physical exercise. The pharmaceutical regimen is reserved for advanced conditions and consists of high-dose calcium and vitamin D supplements, bisphosphonates, and hormonal replacement therapy (HRT). HRT is controversial due to the increased risk of hormone-related cancers and heart disease. Fractures are managed in

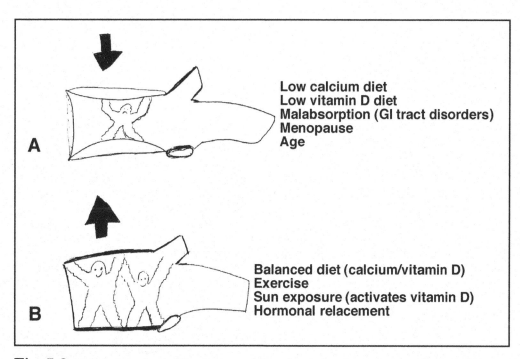

Fig. 5-8 Osteoporosis. A: Biconcave vertebra due to low bone density (osteopenia) as shown with weak trabecula. **B:** Healthy vertebra with normal bone density shown with numerous and strong thick trabecula.

much the same way as in non-osteoporotic patients, but the osteoporosis should be recognized and treated at the same time. Osteoporotic bone heals normally.

Surgical approach. The surgical approach consists of ORIF for most displaced fractures. The added consideration is the need for bone grafting either from iliac bone crest or with synthetic composites.

2. Osteomalacia

In *osteomalacia*, the bone that is present is abnormal due to poor mineralization, and is therefore soft and deformable. Osteomalacia is mainly caused by vitamin D deficiency, which can occur from poor intake, malabsorption, or abnormal or insufficient vitamin D activation. In developed countries the main presentation of osteomalacia is in the elderly, mainly due to dietary insufficiency in vitamin D. Osteomalacia can also occur in children (*rachitism*) but mainly in underdeveloped countries.

Clinical Findings

Osteomalacia can present with general malaise and dull ache in the lower back and thighs. The patients are frequently thin and malnourished.

Simple X-rays show generalized decrease in bone density and also typical band of bone rarefaction called *Looser zone*. The Looser zone represents a healing stress fracture most often seen in the femoral neck or pubic rami. In children with osteomalacia, the long bones are also deformed in varus, and the growth plates are wider than normal due to poor mineralization of newly formed bone. Laboratory tests show elevated alkaline phosphatase from increased osteoblast activity.

Treatment

Conservative approach. Osteomalacia can be successfully treated with vitamin D supplements.

3. Avascular necrosis

Avascular necrosis (AVN) is bone death from ischemia due to lack of blood supply. The most common causes of avascular necrosis are steroid use, alcohol use, pancreatitis, sickle cell anemia, trauma, various metabolic diseases, and drugs. Bones most vulnerable to AVN are the femoral head, the scaphoid bone, the talus, and the proximal humerus.

Clinical Findings

Pain may be either acute or insidious in onset. Joint examination is near normal at the early stage. As the disease progresses, the pain is mechanical and reproducible with manipulation, and ultimately becomes present at rest as the joint architecture is slowly destroyed.

Simple X-ray views of the involved area are ordered. In the early stages, the X-rays may show no abnormality. Early detection of AVN is made possible with MRI, which will detect changes in signal intensity of the bone marrow. AVN is classified into 5 radiographic stages (**Fig. 5-9**).

Treatment

Conservative approach. The primary treatment approach is to stop the offending stimulus, such as lipid lowering drugs or steroids. This option might not always be possible since the drug may be necessary to control other conditions, such as rheumatoid arthritis and lupus. In many situations, the damage is already done and most likely irreversible. One might limit the use of a weight bearing joint or use walking aids. For a non-weight bearing joint like the shoulder, the symptoms might be tolerable and relieved with NSAIDs.

Surgical approach. For a weight-bearing joint like the hip, surgery in the early stages of AVN may save the joint. The surgery consists of restoring blood flow to the femoral head by drilling multiple holes in the subchondral bone with AVN (core decompression). This technique remains controversial with mixed reports for its success.

When the subchondral bone has collapsed, the articular surface becomes incongruent and is ultimately destroyed. The only option then is prosthetic joint replacement (*arthroplasty*).

III. BONE TUMORS

1. Benign bone tumors

Benign bone tumors do not continue to grow over time or do so at an extremely slow rate. Benign bone lesions also do not invade adjacent soft tissues.

2. Malignant bone tumors

Malignant bone tumors are aggressive and can invade the surrounding tissues. They can destroy bone (*osteolytic*) or produce bone (*osteoblastic*). A malignant lesion can originate from bone itself (primary bone neoplasm) or from another type of tissue (metastatic bone lesion). Metastases to bone from breast, prostate, lung, kidney, and thyroid cancers are common. Most metastatic bone lesions are osteolytic. Metastases from breast and prostate can be osteoblastic. Malignant tumors can weaken the bone and increase the risk of fracture (pathologic fracture).

Clinical Findings

The clinical history will reveal how the lesion was discovered (accidentally or investigating for the source of pain), other medical conditions, and family history. The physical findings will reveal the location of the lesion, its tenderness to palpation, and effect on function.

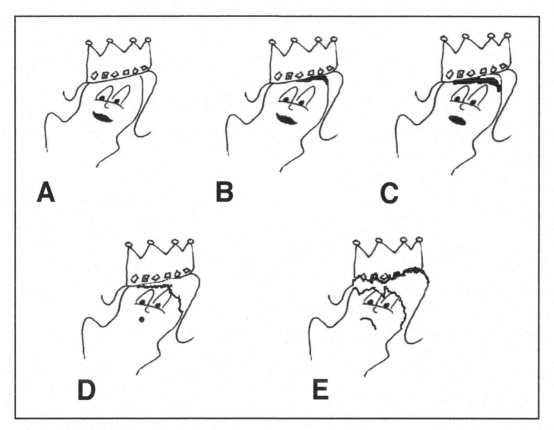

Fig. 5-9 Avascular necrosis stages. A: Stage 1: no visible change on X-ray. **B:** Stage 2: subchondral sclerosis visible on X-ray. **C:** Stage 3: visible subchondral crescent line due to partial revascularization. **D:** Stage 4: subchondral bone collapse. **E:** Stage 5: joint destruction.

Malignant bone lesions may have indolent to severe pain at rest or at night. Pain can increase upon movement of a limb and limit function (limping, stiffness, paralysis from compression of a nerve by an expanding lesion).

Laboratory studies are usually not very informative when investigating for a solitary asymptomatic lesion. Non-specific findings may include chronic anemia and elevated ESR (erythrocyte sedimentation rate) associated with inflammatory conditions.

X-ray views are useful to determine the aggressiveness of the lesion. MRI is used to document the extent of the lesion. A very useful and complementary exam is nuclear bone scan, which gives information about the metabolic activity of the lesion. It also rules out the presence or absence of other lesions (metastases).

When the diagnosis remains unclear, the ultimate diagnostic tool is a biopsy, which can be done by a radiologist using CT guidance or done by an oncologic orthopedic surgeon. The approach to a biopsy is critical and should only be performed with approval of the treating surgeon. An improper biopsy approach may contaminate the biopsy site and jeopardize otherwise healthy tissue, which must then be removed at the time of definitive surgery.

Treatment

Conservative approach. A benign lesion deserves clinical and radiological follow-up to detect any changes. Watchful waiting may be considered for lesions in the bone that do not represent a risk for fracture.

Surgical approach. Surgical management of a benign bone lesion may be indicated if it prevents the normal function of a limb. It usually consists of removing the bony lesion by curettage and filling the bony defect with bone graft. Localized malignant bone tumor should be resected with margins clear of disease to avoid recurrence and to increase the chance for a cure. The surgery involves curettage, debridement and restoration of structural integrity with bone graft or cement, amputation, or limb salvage procedure by resection of the tumor and reconstruction with prosthesis.

CHAPTER 6. PEDIATRIC ORTHOPEDICS

I. FRACTURES AND DISLOCATIONS

A. Anatomy

Most of the growth in children's bones occurs at the growth plates (*physis*), which are located at each extremity of the long bones, and at the distal part of the metacarpal and metatarsal bones. A growth plate is mainly composed of cartilage, which eventually ossifies through the process of mineralization (**Fig. 6-1**). Therefore, growth plates are fragile and can easily break when subjected to trauma. They eventually close at puberty, once growth has finished, under hormonal influence. Compared with adult bone, a child's bone is more flexible and can bend to a certain extent before breaking. The bone-laying matrix (*periosteum*) is also much thicker.

B. Approach

When seeing a child who has suffered an injury, parents are often upset and need appropriate reassurance. Therefore, a gentle and reassuring approach is best. When addressing an injury, it is extremely important to document the circumstances under which the injury occurred. If the child is calm, complete your history and start your examination without disturbing the child. However, a proper examination requires exposure of the injured area and mandates uncovering the child, so gently proceed despite any explosive tantrums.

For the physical exam, follow the systematic "**I** Personally **M**ake **S**ure and **C**heck" approach (cf. Chapter 1, General Approach):

1. **I**nspection
2. **P**alpation
3. **M**obility (active and passive range of motion)
4. **S**pecific maneuvers
5. **C**omplementary exam

The examination may require the help of a parent or an orderly to restrain the child. Capture the child's attention with toys if any are available, and carry out the examination with assurance. Your calm, confident manner will greatly reassure the anxious parents.

Radiological examinations may reveal a fracture or dislocation. In addition to the fracture patterns seen in adults, in the pediatric population, a fracture can also occur through a growth plate (**Fig. 6-2**). An impaction fracture involving the growth plate (*Salter-Harris V*) has the worst prognosis for growth arrest due to complete de-

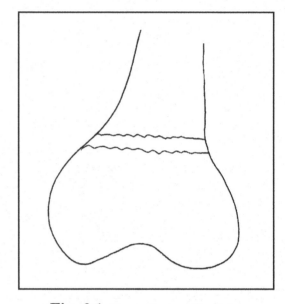

Fig. 6-1 Normal growth plate.

struction of the growth plate. The greenstick type fracture is frequent in children, since the soft cortical bone breaks under tension, but may only deform on the side receiving the pressure (compression) of the trauma (**Fig. 6-3**).

Treatment

Conservative approach. Non-displaced fractures can be immobilized with a cast for 4 to 6 weeks. Slightly displaced fractures can be reduced in the ER under mild sedation, or in the OR under general anesthesia. Cast immobilization should follow for the same period of time.

Surgical approach. A greenstick fracture can be reduced under sedation in the ER or under general anesthesia in the operating room under general anesthesia. Due to the elastic recoil of this type of fracture, the orthopedic surgeon may overcorrect the fracture and break the remaining intact cortex to achieve an anatomic reduction. The broken limb is then immobilized in a cast.

Displaced intra-articular fractures require open anatomic reduction and internal fixation (ORIF). Particular attention is paid to the growth plate to avoid complications, such as partial or complete growth arrest of the growth plate, which could lead to angulation or length discrepancies.

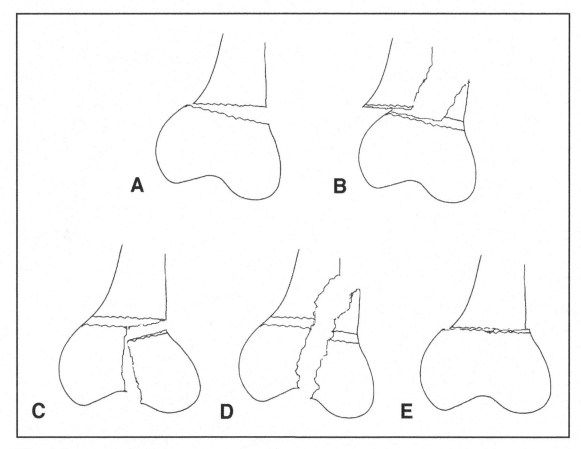

Fig. 6-2 Growth plate fractures (Salter Harris classification). A: Complete fracture through the growth plate (Salter Harris I). **B:** Fracture through the growth plate with extension to the metaphysis (Salter Harris II). **C:** Fracture through the growth plate, with extension to the epiphysis (Salter Harris III). **D:** Fracture passing through the epiphysis, growth plate and metaphysis (Salter Harris IV). **E:** Impaction fracture with collapse of the growth plate (Salter Harris V).

C. Specific Problems

1. Radial head dislocation or "pulled elbow"

Radial head dislocation is a classic injury in the pediatric population. It occurs when an adult suddenly pulls on the arm of a child (**Fig. 6-4**). This injury is most often a subluxation rather than a complete dislocation of the radial head.

Clinical Findings

The child experiences intense sudden pain. The elbow is locked in slight flexion with forearm pronation. The patient often guards the elbow and refuses to use the arm. The elbow may be swollen and tender on palpation over the radial head.

Simple X-rays of the elbow joint can be overlooked as normal. If there is any doubt, consult with a radiologist for an expert opinion, since radial head dislocations can be subtle and missed.

Treatment

Conservative approach. The radial head can usually be reduced with gentle supination of the child's hand while gradually flexing the elbow and applying gentle pressure with your thumb over the radial head. The child can wear a sling for a few days for comfort.

Surgical approach. The surgical approach is never necessary for a true pulled elbow.

2. Slipped capital femoral epiphysis

Slipped capital femoral epiphysis implies displacement of the proximal femoral epiphysis from its normal position (**Fig. 6-5**) to a posterolateral position relative to the femoral neck. This condition occurs secondarily to

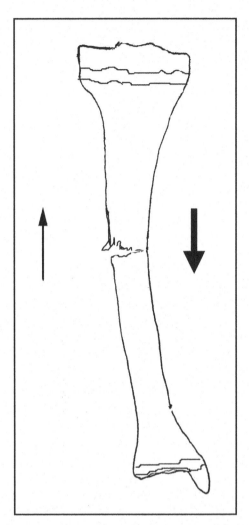

Fig. 6-3 Greenstick fracture. Incomplete fracture with failure of the cortex on the tension side (thin arrow) and deformation of the cortex on the compression side (thick arrow).

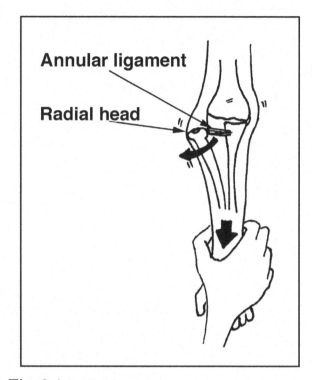

Fig. 6-4 Radial head dislocation. With sudden pull on the arm (thick black arrow), the radial head dislocates (curved black arrow) by slipping out of the annular ligament. Reduction is possible with gentle traction on the arm, pressure on the radial head, supination and flexion of the elbow.

an imbalance between growth hormone and sex hormones during adolescence. During this time, the growth plate of the proximal femur is still fragile, and the increasing weight of the growing adolescent may cause a progressive displacement of the epiphysis or a sudden acute displacement.

Clinical Findings

Common symptoms are vague pain referred to the knee and limping. Common signs are atrophy of the thigh, shortening and external rotation of the involved leg, and weakness of the hip abductors.

Simple X-rays of the involved hip are diagnostic. The femoral epiphysis slipping off the neck is analogous to a scoop of ice cream slipping along an ice cream cone

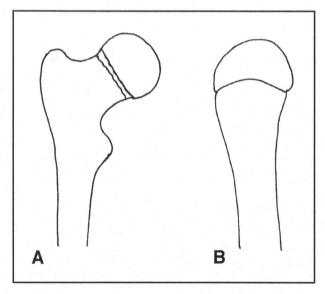

Fig. 6-5 Normal pediatric hip. A: AP view. **B:** Lateral view.

(**Fig. 6-6**). The investigation should include X-rays of the opposite hip, since 25% of adolescent patients can have bilateral slip of the epiphysis. A bone scan can detect abnormal activity at the proximal hip growth plate in radiographically occult cases.

Complementary tests include studies to rule out metabolic diseases, such as chronic renal failure, endocrinopathies, and hypothyroidism.

There are 2 main complications due to this condition: chondrolysis (thinning of the cartilage) and *avascular necrosis* (AVN) of the femoral head.

Treatment

Conservative approach. Nowadays, there is no room for a conservative treatment for this condition. The treatment consisted mainly in immobilization in a cast that includes the waist and involved leg (spica immobilization) for 6 to 8 weeks. Follow-up X-rays were done every 6 months until skeletal maturity to assess healing.

Surgical approach. In situ pinning of the femoral head (**Fig. 6-7**) to prevent further slipping and accelerate fusion of the femoral head growth plate (*epiphysiodesis*) is the treatment of choice in all cases.

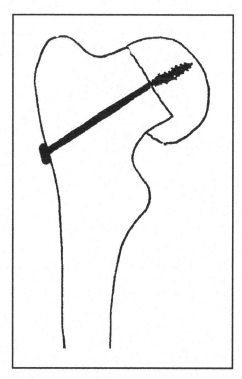

Fig. 6-7 In situ pinning. No attempt is made to correct the deformation to avoid further damage and complication, such as avascular necrosis. The screw is inserted aiming at the center of the femoral head.

3. Congenital hip dislocation

From birth to the first 6 months of life, the proximal femoral head is soft and fits loosely within the acetabulum. It is therefore at risk of dislocation. Congenital hip dislocation often occurs in breech babies (20%) and is more common in females. All newborn babies are screened for hip dislocation by the pediatrician before discharge from the ward.

Clinical Findings. In order for you to perform a good physical exam, the baby must be calm, since muscle contraction could mask the dislocation. Have the baby fully undressed and supine on a firm mattress. Up to the age of 3 months, few clinical signs such as limited abduction, buttock skin fold asymmetry or leg length discrepancy are present. The diagnosis is mainly made using specific maneuvers.

The specific maneuvers to diagnose an unstable hip are the *Ortolani* (reduction) (**Fig. 6-8**) and the *Barlow* (provocative) signs (**Fig. 6-9**). A mild physiologic laxity is often found (subluxable hip) up to the age of 3 months but should disappear thereafter.

After the first 3 months, the classical findings of a congenital hip dislocation such as limited abduction, leg

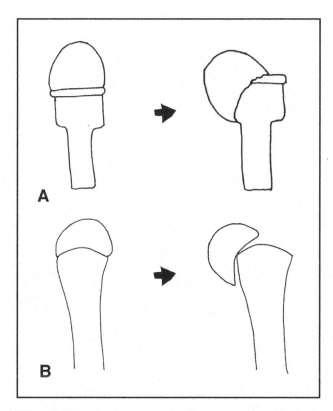

Fig. 6-6 Ice cream cone analogy. A: Ice cream ball slipping along the side of a cone. **B:** Lateral view of a femoral epiphysis that slips from the femoral neck.

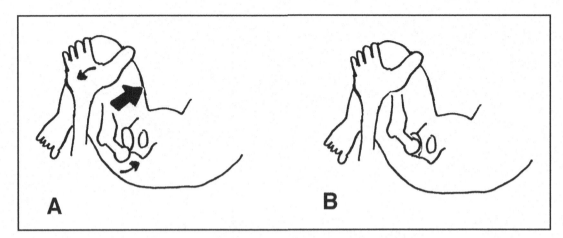

Fig. 6-8 Ortolani sign. A: The examiner exerts an upward force (thick black arrow) with a twist (thin black arrow) to reduce the dislocated hip. **B:** The Ortolani sign is positive when the hip reduces with the maneuver. A negative Ortolani sign may imply that the hip is in a fixed dislocation position and cannot be reduced with the maneuver.

length discrepancy (*Galleazzi sign*) and skin fold asymmetry are usually present. Past the walking age, limping due to unilateral dislocation or waddling due bilateral dislocation are noticeable.

To help confirm and better plan the treatment, the ultrasound has become the ultimate diagnostic tool for babies up to the age of 6 months. It can be done to examine the hip structures without movement (statically) and also with motion of the hip (dynamically). Simple X-rays are not sensitive in that period of time since the femoral head is almost entirely made of cartilage and not clearly visible. In an older child with a normal hip, the femoral head ossification center should be within the infero-medial quadrant of the *Perkin / Hilgenreiner quadrant* (**Fig. 6-10**) on the X-ray of the pelvis.

Treatment

Conservative approach. *Clinical suspicion of an unstable or dislocated hip in a newborn or older child warrants an urgent referral to a pediatric orthopedic surgeon.*

While physiologic hip laxity regresses spontaneously in most babies by the age of 3 months without further treatment, hip dislocation or "dislocatable" hips will require treatment with special harness or abduction brace (*Pavlick harness*). Casting is used to keep the hip in place once a closed reduction has been performed under general anesthesia following failure of the harness. Forced reduction should never be attempted due to the risk of avascular necrosis of the femoral head.

Surgical approach. Surgery is indicated when the hip is locked in a dislocated position. Open reduction is performed. A femoral osteotomy might be needed in an older child (>18 months) to reposition the femoral head within the acetabulum. When there is significant acetabular dysplasia, a pelvic osteotomy is done to rotate the acetabulum and restore a "roof" above the femoral head.

4. Osteochondrosis (Osgood-Schlatter and Sever diseases)

Ostechondrosis is a condition that relates to tendon insertions on secondary ossification centers (SOC)

Fig. 6-9 Barlow sign. With a downward pressure on the knee (thick black arrow) and a twist (thin black arrow), the unstable hip dislocates easily. The hip usually spontaneously reduces upon pressure release.

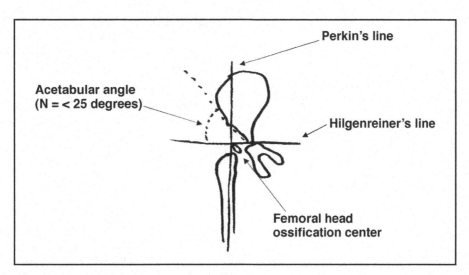

Fig. 6-10 Perkin/Hilgenreiner quadrant. A quadrant is drawn over the X-ray of the pelvis. The femoral head ossification center should be within the infero-medial quadrant for normal development. If the ossification center is situated anywhere else, the hip may be dislocated. The acetabular dysplasia can be documented with the acetabular angle, which should normally be less than 25 degrees.

or apophysis. SOCs are similar to epiphyses but are not part of a joint. These "little growth plates" are fragile when loaded under tension (**Fig. 6-11**). When children increase their activity level and mass, they can put significant tension on the tendon and their SOCs. Fast growth at puberty can also increase tension on SOCs.

The most frequent sites of inflammation are the patellar tendon insertion at the tibial tuberosity (*Osgood-Schlatter disease*) and the Achilles tendon insertion on the calcaneum (*Sever disease*). The children will complain of pain mostly during their physical activity but pain may occur at rest in more severe cases.

Clinical Findings

On inspection, the tendon insertion may appear swollen. There is localized pain on palpation that is exacerbated with passive and active motion.

Simple X-rays are usually normal but may reveal an avulsed SOC.

Treatment

Conservative approach. The child is advised to switch from extreme sports to milder activity levels. NSAIDs, ice, and physical therapy can help with pain management. Once the inflammation has subsided, stretching exercises of the involved musculo-tendinous unit(s) will prevent recurrence. In more extreme cases, cast immobilization may be indicated for 4 to 6 weeks, especially if the SOC is slightly displaced (<1cm).

Surgical approach. Operative measures are rarely, if ever, indicated. Acute traumatic avulsion of an apophysis with displacement more than 1 cm is treated like a fracture and requires ORIF (**Fig. 6-12**). A painful loose ossicle deep in the patellar tendon will be treated by surgical excision at maturity.

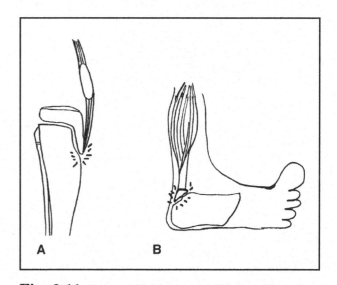

Fig. 6-11 Osgood-Schlatter and Sever diseases. A: Tension of the patellar tendon on the tibial tuberosity causes stress on the underlying growth plate (Osgood-Schlatter disease). **B:** Tension of the Achilles tendon on the calcaneum secondary ossification center (SOC) causes osteochondritis (Sever disease).

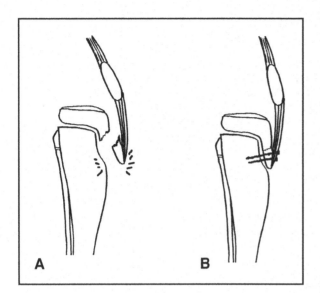

Fig. 6-12 SOC fracture. A: Avulsion of the tibial tuberosity. **B:** ORIF of the tibial tuberosity.

5. Osteogenesis Imperfecta (brittle bone disease)

Osteogenesis imperfecta (OI) means imperfect bone formation. It is a condition due to a genetic mutation that causes a deficient production (not enough) or a defective protein in the making of type I collagen. Type I collagen is also found in ligaments, teeth, and the sclera of the eyes. As a result, all of these constituents are fragile. OI is autosomal dominant, meaning that a parent with the disease has a 50 percent chance to have a child with OI. The symptoms and disability may vary. If neither parent of a child with OI has OI, it implies that the genetic defect is secondary to a spontaneous mutation.

Clinical Findings

Individuals with OI may have different clinical characteristics of the disease. Besides brittle bones, other features include short stature, a triangular face, respiratory problems, and hearing loss.

There are 4 main types of OI:

Type I has a normal collagen structure. It is therefore the mildest form of OI and also the most common. The collagen is normal but is present in a smaller quantity than normal. The bones are fragile and break easily. Bone deformities are less frequent. Associated features are bluish sclera of the eyes, and the teeth are more prone to cavities.

Type II has abnormal collagen structure, which predispose the bones to break even while the fetus is in the womb. It is the most severe type. An affected child can die at birth.

Type III is also a severe form of OI. Features of this type are short stature, fragile teeth, spinal deformities, and respiratory complications. Children are often born with fractures.

Type IV involves abnormal collagen, but is moderately severe in its presentation. The sclera is normal, and bone deformities are mild. Children with this type are usually shorter than average and have fragile teeth.

The incidence of fractures usually decreases as the child matures. However, the bone may become fragile again with menopause or in old age.

Treatment

Conservative approach. Most fractures will be treated with casting or bracing to allow bone healing. Movement and weight bearing are encouraged as soon as possible to compensate for the long periods of immobilization that can demineralize bone.

Surgical approach. Indications for surgery are repeated fractures, deformity, and non-union. Long bone fractures can be treated with intramedullary nailing. Special nails can elongate as the bone grows, like a telescope. Spinal fusion is indicated for significant deformation of the spine, mainly to avoid cardio-pulmonary complications.

6. Child abuse

The possibility of child abuse must be considered for all fractures of long bones occurring before the walking stage. After carefully documenting the history with regard to mechanism of injury, timing and the possible individual(s) involved, perform a detailed physical examination.

Clinical Findings

Look for the presence of hematomas, burns, and bruises. A retinal exam may reveal hemorrhage of the retina due to shaking. X-rays of the site of injury should be ordered. If you have any doubt, do a complete work-up, which includes a complete radiological skeletal survey to identify other fracture sites.

Any long bone fractures, especially the metaphyseal-epiphyseal fracture (corner fracture or bucket-handle fractures) in children not yet walking, as well as rib and spine fractures are suspicious for child abuse. A CT scan of the brain will diagnose cerebral hematoma.

Treatment

Hospitalization is required to conduct a full inquiry. The social service team must be involved to inquire about socio-economic environment. The hospital probably has a multi-disciplinary team that is responsible for investigating possible cases of child abuse. This team should be alerted.

II. OTHER PEDIATRIC CONDITIONS

A. Legg-Calve-Perthes Disease (Hip Osteonecrosis)

Legg-Calve-Perthes disease is an idiopathic *osteonecrosis* (bone avascular necrosis) of the proximal femoral epiphysis. It usually occurs between the ages of 3 and 11. During this time, changes in the vascular supply of the femoral head may occur, and the femoral head becomes vulnerable to inflammation and trauma, which can cause ischemia. Boys are affected 5 times more often than girls.

Clinical Findings

Common symptoms are limping and pain. Common signs are atrophy of the thigh of the involved leg and limited range of motion. The abduction can be less than 20 degrees and there may be a hip contracture (*hip flexum*).

The age of the patient is the most important prognostic factor; the older the child when the disease appears, the worse the prognosis. The natural history of the disease is such that the femoral center of ossification will first become avascular, then fragment into many pieces, and eventually heal, often in a nonspherical shape.

Radiographic evaluation should include simple X-rays of the pelvis in the AP view, and also lateral in the frog leg position. The osteonecrosis of the femoral epiphysis can be partial or complete (**Fig. 6-13**).

Complementary exams can include a bone scan when the symptoms are present, but the X-rays are unremarkable. MRI can also evaluate the vascular status of the femoral head.

Treatment

Conservative approach. In patients less than 6 years of age, there is a good chance that the femoral head will recover and remain relatively spherical after resolution of the disease. After the age of 6, the prognosis is uncertain, and mainly depends on the extent of femoral head involvement with necrosis, fragmentation, and ultimately, healing, and remodeling.

Young patients can therefore be treated with physiotherapy to restore and maintain the range of motion. For older children, the main treatment principle is to keep the femoral head contained within the acetabulum to help preserve its spherical shape. This goal might be achieved by physiotherapy and soft tissue release (adductor tenotomy), and or the wear of a brace or cast that holds the hip in abduction. The cast is worn 6 weeks while the brace is discontinued when there are radiographic signs of re-ossification. Uncontained within the acetabulum, the femoral head will become flat (*coxa plana*) and enlarged (*coxa magna*) (**Fig. 6-14**).

Surgical approach. The surgical option for containment of the femoral head is to perform either a pelvic osteotomy, a femoral osteotomy or both to provide more coverage of the femoral head and protection against possible deformation. It is however essential to first restore an adequate range of motion of the hip prior to any osteotomy as such surgical procedure done on a stiff hip might end in "catastrophy".

B. Lower Limb Alignment Anomalies

The mechanical axis of the lower limb goes through the center of the femoral head, the center of the tibial plateau,

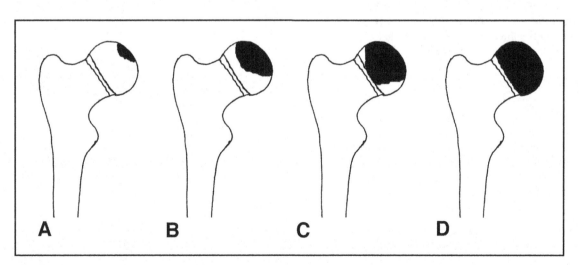

Fig. 6-13 Legg-Calve-Perthes disease. A: Minimal osteonecrosis. **B:** Less than half of the epiphysis is affected. **C:** More than half of the epiphysis is affected. **D:** The entire epiphysis is osteonecrotic.

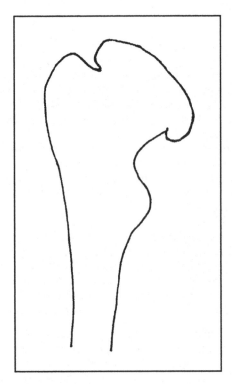

Fig. 6-14 Legg-Calve-Perthes disease sequel. Illustration showing coxa plana (flat head) and coxa magna (enlarged head) of the femoral head.

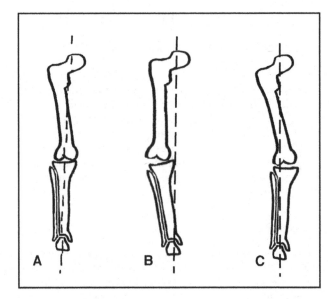

Fig. 6-15 Mechanical axis. AP view of the right leg. **A:** Normal mechanical alignment with the mechanical axis passing through the center of the femoral head, the center of the tibial plateau, and the center of the ankle. **B:** Genu varum with the mechanical axis passing medial to the knee. **C:** Genu valgum with the mechanical axis passing lateral to the knee.

and the center of the ankle joint (**Fig. 6-15A**). Lower limb alignment can be grossly determined by holding a string or rope over the femoral pulse, which is approximately over the femoral head, and stretching it down over the ankle joint. If the center of the knee largely passes lateral to the rope, the limb alignment is in *genu varum* (**Fig. 6-15B**). If the center of the knee passes medial to the rope, the alignment is in *genu valgum* (**Fig. 6-15C**).

1. Genu varum

Newborn babies normally have lower limb alignment in genu varum, which corrects itself progressively until 2 years of age. In underdeveloped countries, a common cause of persistent genu varum is vitamin D deficiency (rickets) from malnutrition.

Clinical Findings

Genu varum can be documented by measuring the space between the femoral condyles. To do so, the baby is held supine with the leg stretched and ankles touching.

Simple X-rays that view the complete lower limb are helpful to calculate precisely the deformity, but are usually not indicated until the age of 18 months.

Treatment

Conservative approach. Genu varum in young children usually resolves spontaneously. Close follow-up is recommended.

Surgical approach. Physiologic genu varum does not require treatment. In persistent genu varum, one must rule out a metabolic disease (rickets) or growth abnormality (*Blount's disease*- tibia vara) or a skeletal dysplasia (*achondroplasia*). Surgical correction of persistent genu varum consists of either partial epiphysiodesis of the lateral growth plate or osteotomy of the proximal tibia, whenever indicated.

2. Genu valgum

Genu valgum is common from the age of 2 to the age of 5, and usually corrects spontaneously by the age of 7.

Clinical Findings

The genu valgum can be measured by the space between medial malleoli when the patient is lying down or standing with the inside of the knees touching. A 4 cm gap at 4 years old is normal. When a significant genu valgum is present (10 cm), a full diagnostic work-up must be done to rule out metabolic anomalies or skeletal dysplasia. The familial morphotype may explain a persistent genu valgum in some teenagers.

Treatment

Conservative approach. Clinical follow-up once a year is appropriate to reassure the child and parents, since the majority of patients will correct spontaneously. The distance between the internal malleoli is measured for the record.

Surgical approach. With a persistent distance between the medial malleoli of 10 cm or more, after the age of 11 in girls and 12 in boys, the surgeon can consider provoking a partial growth arrest (*epiphysiodesis*) on the medial side of the growth plate to obtain a spontaneous correction of the genu valgum. However, this technique is imprecise and may partially correct the deformity. If done after the age of 12 in girls and 13 in boys, a more precise technique is to perform an osteotomy. The osteotomy is usually done on the bone with most deformity (distal femur or proximal tibia).

3. Axial rotation (toe-in, toe-out)

Many parents will be concerned with the direction the feet of their child are pointing to, especially when pointing inward (toe-in) and pointing outward (toe-out).

Clinical Findings. The levels at which the malrotation is occurring can be determined with a good physical exam, which will focus on the hips, the knees, and the feet. Asymmetry can be a sign of an organic condition.

To rule out malrotation that originates at the hip level, examine the patient lying flat on the abdomen. The legs are flexed 90 degrees at the knees, and the feet are left to drop outward in internal rotation at the hip joint, and inward in external rotation for comparison (**Fig. 6-16**). Another way to explain normal femoral anteversion (forward displacement) is to visualize the hip joint from a bird's eye view (**Fig. 6-17**).

To rule out malrotation that originates at the tibial level, continue the exam with the patient flat on the abdomen. The knees are flexed at 90 degrees and the axis of the tibia is assessed. Normally the axis going through the malleoli should be parallel or divergent, which implies slight external tibial torsion (**Fig. 6-18**).

To rule out malrotation alignment originating from the feet, look at the plantar surface of the feet and place a pen or stick by the lateral side of the foot. The majority of the lateral surface of the foot should fall flat against the surface of the pen (**Fig. 6-19**).

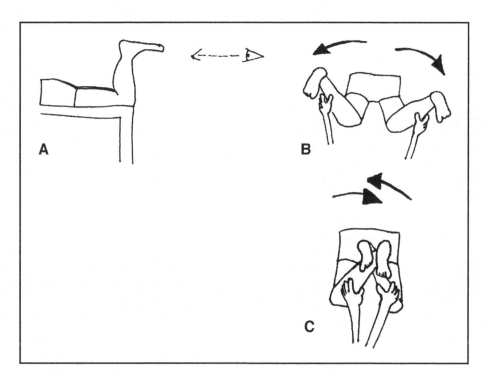

Fig. 6-16 Testing for femur malrotation. A: The patient is prone on abdomen with knees flexed 90 degrees. **B:** Exam of internal rotation at the hip level. **C:** Exam of external rotation at the hip level.

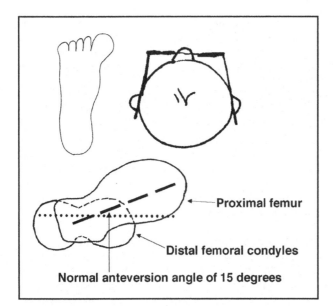

Fig. 6-17 Normal femoral anteversion. To better visualize normal femoral anteversion, look at the patient with a bird's eye view. The axis of the femoral head (thick dashed line) is angulated anteriorly (in anteversion) relative to the axis of the distal femoral condyles (dotted line). Normal anteversion is about 15 degrees.

Toe-in

The hip joint can be responsible for in-toeing due to a torsional deformity of the proximal femur. With the patient lying prone on the abdomen and knees flexed at 90 degrees, the feet can spontaneously drop flat sideways (**Fig. 6-20**). Excessive internal rotation at the hip joint with respect to external rotation signifies that the femoral neck has too much anteversion (**Fig. 6-21**). Femoral anteversion may result from sitting in the "W-sitting" position with feet outward on each side of the hips (**Fig. 6-22**).

The tibia can also cause in-toeing due to a torsional deformity. When the axes of the malleoli form an angle that points posterior to the heels, there is definite internal tibial torsion (**Fig. 6-23**). Excessive internal tibial rotation can be due to the intrauterine position of the child and therefore is present at birth. It should spontaneously disappear with growth. Internal tibial torsion can persist due to the child sleeping in a fetal position or from the habit of sitting on his or her heels.

In-toeing as a deformity of the foot may be due to metatarsal bone deviation in varus relative to the hindfoot; so-called *metatarsus adductus*. Metatarsus adductus (**Fig. 6-24**) is a benign condition and should be easily reducible with gentle pressure over the forefoot (**Fig. 6-25**). When the pressure is released, the foot bounces back to its deformed status. A fixed deformation

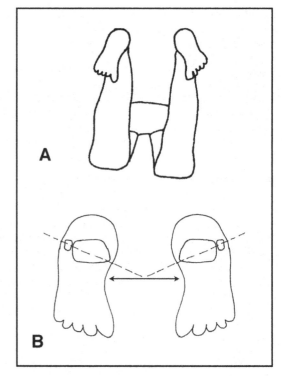

Fig. 6-18 Assessment of tibial malrotation. **A:** The patient is prone on the abdomen with the knees flexed 90 degrees. **B:** Note the axis of the malleoli (dashed lines) by placing a pen or stick on the plantar surface of the foot as trying to connect both internal and external malleoli. The axes should be parallel or intersect each other at a wide angle at the level of the plantar arch of both feet (black double arrow).

(not reducible) may indicate more serious conditions, such as neuromuscular or congenital pathologies, and must be ruled out by a pediatric orthopedic surgeon. If there is any doubt, the parents are better off going home reassured than consulting too late for a deformity that is now fixed and requires a surgical approach.

Toe-out

Excessive out-toeing is also a cause of concern for the parents. The causes are the precise opposites of causes in-toeing. At the hip level, out-toeing is due to femoral neck retroversion, which is identified by the lack of internal rotation. With the child lying flat on the abdomen with the knees flexed at 90 degrees, the feet will not spontaneously drop on each side on the body (**Fig. 6-26**).

At the tibial level, out-toeing can be caused by excessive external tibial torsion. With the child lying flat on the abdomen and knees flexed 90 degrees, the axes going through the malleoli will form an angle with the summit pointing to the big toes (**Fig. 6-27**).

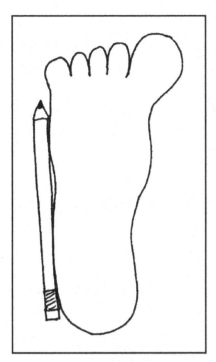

Fig. 6-19 Assessment of foot malalignment.
Looking at the plantar surface of the foot, place a pen or pencil along the lateral side of the plantar surface. Most of the lateral side of the foot should come in contact with the surface of the pen or pencil.

Out-toeing at the foot level is most frequently due to loss of the plantar arch, such as flat foot deformity. A flexible flat foot deformity means that the longitudinal arch of the foot is restored when the foot is held in a non-weight bearing position (**Fig. 6-28**). This condition is usually asymptomatic. The subtalar motion and ankle

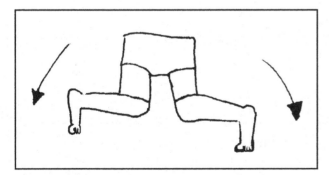

Fig. 6-20 Increased femoral neck anteversion.
The patient is prone on the abdomen with knees flexed 90 degrees. Increased femoral neck anteversion will spontaneously cause an exaggerated capability to internally rotate the hip. External rotation will be decreased.

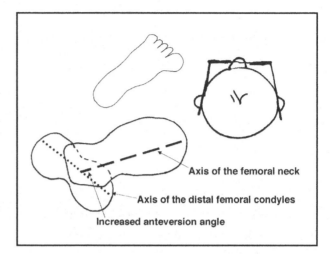

Fig. 6-21 In-toeing from increased hip anteversion. To better visualize abnormal femoral anteversion causing in-toeing, look at the patient with a bird's eye view. The axis of the femoral neck (thick dashed line) is angulated anteriorly (in anteversion) relative to the axis of the distal femoral condyles (dotted line). An abnormally anteverted hip joint will affect the rotation of the whole limb, causing in-toeing of the foot.

dorsiflexion are normal. Whenever the subtalar motion is limited or dorsiflexion is restricted by a tight heel cord, or the plantar arch is not restored with non-weight bearing, the child must be referred to a pediatric orthopedic surgeon to rule out congenital or neuromuscular conditions. A flexible flatfoot deformity may also be the consequence of a persistent genu valgum.

Treatment

Conservative approach. The vast majority of lower limb malalignment in the infant will resolve spontaneously or with the help of preventive measures. Long-

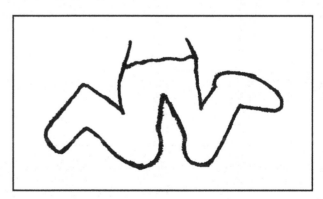

Fig. 6-22 W sitting position.

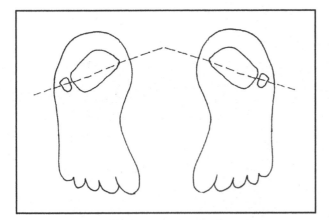

Fig. 6-23 Increased internal tibial torsion. Feet plantar view with knees flexed 90 degrees. The axes of the malleoli (dashed lines) of both tibiae are forming a summit angle close to the heels, indicating abnormal internal tibial torsion. The examiner should not pay attention to the feet when looking for abnormal tibial torsion, since they may look like they are pointing straight.

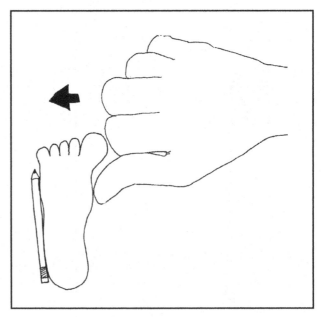

Fig. 6-25 Flexible metatarsus adductus. A physiologic metatarsus adductus should be reducible with gentle pressure over the forefoot.

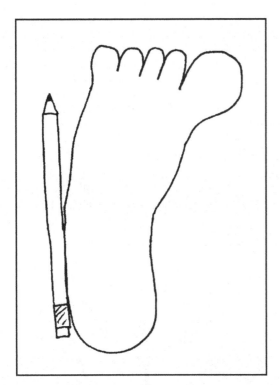

Fig. 6-24 Metatarsus adductus. Right foot plantar view. When pressing a pen or pencilalong the side of the foot only partial contact is obtained, with most of the forefoot off the pen or pencil.

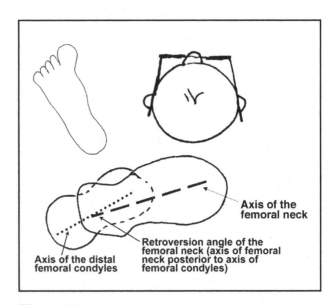

Fig. 6-26 Out-toeing from hip retroversion. To better visualize abnormal femoral retroversion causing out-toeing, look at the patient with a bird's eye view. The axis of the femoral head (thick dashed line) is angulated posteriorly (in retroversion) relative to the axis of the distal femoral condyles (dotted line). An abnormally retroverted hip joint will affect the rotation of the whole limb, causing out-toeing of the foot.

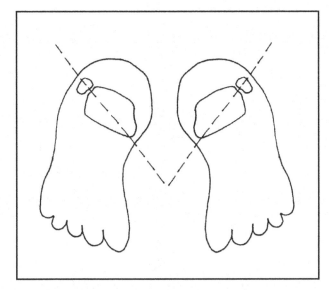

Fig. 6-27 Increased external tibial torsion. With the patient prone on the abdomen and knees flexed 90 degrees, look at the feet's plantar surface. Using a pen or stick, the examiner can make the axes of the malleoli (dashed lines) of both tibiae form an angle with the summit pointing to the big toes, indicating abnormal internal tibial torsion. The examiner should not pay attention to the feet when looking for abnormal tibial torsion, since they may look like they are pointing straight.

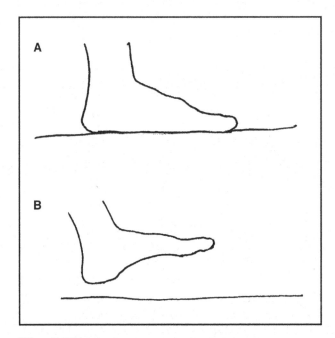

Fig. 6-28 Flexible flat foot. A: With weight-bearing, the plantar arch is flattened. **B:** With non-weight-bearing position, the plantar arch appears normal.

term correction will occur with growth. A good sleeping position for an infant is on the back or on the side. For toddlers, the main preventive measure is to adopt good sitting habits, avoiding a pattern of sitting with exaggerated lower limb deformation.

For in-toeing, no orthosis has proven to be effective in correcting femoral anteversion. However, if the internal tibial torsion persists after the age of 18 months despite good positional control, a nocturnal bar (*Dennis Browne*) can be used as prescribed by the pediatric orthopedic surgeon.

For asymptomatic out-toeing due to a flexible flat foot (age 2 and 5 years), reassurance is key. Arch support orthoses are not indicated. For the symptomatic patient with normal test results, arch support may provide relief.

Surgical approach. The indications for the correction of misaligned lower limbs are failure of a deformity to spontaneously correct itself with growth, the presence of a grossly asymmetric deformity, aggravating symptoms, and symptomatic congenital or evolving neuromuscular conditions. The surgery is tailored and aimed at restoring the proper mechanical axis to the lower limb.

C. Scoliosis

Scoliosis is characterized by a misalignment of the spine, as seen when looking at an individual face to face (frontal view) (**Fig. 6-29**). A scoliosis can be postural (secondary to pain or difference in leg length) or structural, which is characterized by deformed vertebrae and soft tissue contractures.

Scoliosis can be classified according to the age of the patient (infantile 0 to 3 years, juvenile 3 to 12, and adolescent). The deformity can be localized mainly in the

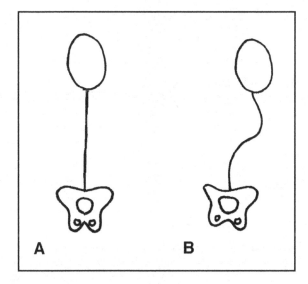

Fig. 6-29 Scoliosis. A: AP view of a normal spine. **B:** AP view of a spine with scoliosis.

thoracic, the thoraco-lumbar, or the lumbar area. The most frequent cause of scoliosis is idiopathic (65%), congenital (15%), and due to neuromuscular diseases (10%). There might also be a family history of scoliosis.

Clinical Findings

Pain is rarely a symptom of scoliosis. A painful thoraco-lumbar spine usually results as a long-term sequella of scoliosis and is mostly seen in the adult population. An extreme deformity can ultimately cause cardiopulmonary insufficiency from mechanical compromise or spinal cord compression with neurological deficits.

The physical exam is done standing behind the patient. The patient's back should be completely revealed.

With the patient standing and then bending forward with hands held together, carry out the following examination.

1. Inspection: i)   shoulder height asymmetry
             ii) protruding shoulder blade
             iii) waist fold asymmetry
             iv) pelvis tilt
             v)   when bending forward, the spinal deformity will appear, creating an asymmetric hump due to malrotation of the vertebrae.

2. Palpation: the spine is usually not painful to palpation

3. Mobility (active and passive range of motion)

4. Specific maneuver:
   i) *String test:* Holding a string with a small weight hanging can help detect the translation or shift of the trunk. The string is held over the C7 spinous process and allowed to drop straight down. It should normally fall aligned with the gluteal fold. With a scoliotic spine, the string would fall on either side of the gluteal fold.
   ii) Full neurological exam is mandatory.

5. Complementary exams:
Simple AP and lateral X-rays will permit measurement of the deformity. The angle of each curvature is documented by measuring the *Cobb angle* (**Fig. 6-30**). The pelvic X-ray can give an approximation of bone maturity with the *Risser sign* (**Fig. 6-31**).

Treatment

All children with a scoliotic spine should be referred to a specialist for in-depth primary assessment.

Conservative approach. A progressive structural idiopathic scoliosis in the adolescent requires treatment. Physiotherapy cannot correct the spinal deformity, but braces can help stabilize the deformity until skeletal maturity.

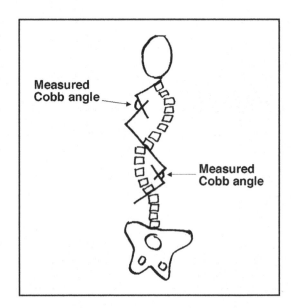

Fig. 6-30 Cobb angle. Lines from the upper and lower vertebral bodies of a curvature are drawn. Perpendicular lines are drawn such that the upper line and lower line at each end of a curvature will intersect. The resulting angle is measured to obtain the angle of the deformity.

Surgical approach. Indications for surgical intervention in scoliosis include documented progression of the curvature, or unusual etiology (e.g., tumor related). The surgery involves straightening of the spine using metal rods, and arthrodesis between vertebral bodies to permanently fix the spine.

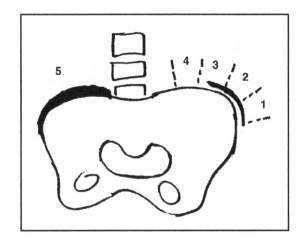

Fig. 6-31 Risser sign. The Risser sign reveals bone maturation. A completely fused iliac crest apophysis (thick black line, Risser 5) is an indication of skeletal maturity. With growth the iliac apophysis (thin black line in the numbered area, Risser 3) progressively fuses with the iliac wing.

INDEX

INDEX

RAPID LEARNING AND RETENTION THROUGH THE MEDMASTER SERIES:

CLINICAL NEUROANATOMY MADE RIDICULOUSLY SIMPLE, by S. Goldberg
CLINICAL BIOCHEMISTRY MADE RIDICULOUSLY SIMPLE, by S. Goldberg
CLINICAL ANATOMY MADE RIDICULOUSLY SIMPLE, by S. Goldberg
CLINICAL PHYSIOLOGY MADE RIDICULOUSLY SIMPLE, by S. Goldberg
CLINICAL MICROBIOLOGY MADE RIDICULOUSLY SIMPLE, by M. Gladwin and B. Trattler
CLINICAL PHARMACOLOGY MADE RIDICULOUSLY SIMPLE, by J.M. Olson
OPHTHALMOLOGY MADE RIDICULOUSLY SIMPLE, by S. Goldberg
PSYCHIATRY MADE RIDICULOUSLY SIMPLE, by W.V. Good and J. Nelson
CLINICAL PSYCHOPHARMACOLOGY MADE RIDICULOUSLY SIMPLE, by J. Preston and J. Johnson
USMLE STEP 1 MADE RIDICULOUSLY SIMPLE, by A. Carl
USMLE STEP 2 MADE RIDICULOUSLY SIMPLE, by A. Carl
USMLE STEP 3 MADE RIDICULOUSLY SIMPLE, by A. Carl
BEHAVIORAL MEDICINE MADE RIDICULOUSLY SIMPLE, by F. Seitz and J. Carr
ACID-BASE, FLUIDS, AND ELECTROLYTES MADE RIDICULOUSLY SIMPLE, by R. Preston
THE FOUR-MINUTE NEUROLOGIC EXAM, by S. Goldberg
MEDICAL SPANISH MADE RIDICULOUSLY SIMPLE, by T. Espinoza-Abrams
CLINICAL ANATOMY AND PHYSIOLOGY FOR THE ANGRY HEALTH PROFESSIONAL, by J.V. Stewart
PREPARING FOR MEDICAL PRACTICE MADE RIDICULOUSLY SIMPLE, by D.M. Lichtstein
MED'TOONS (260 humorous medical cartoons by the author) by S. Goldberg
CLINICAL RADIOLOGY MADE RIDICULOUSLY SIMPLE, by H. Ouellette and P. Tétreault
NCLEX-RN MADE RIDICULOUSLY SIMPLE, by A. Carl
THE PRACTITIONER'S POCKET PAL: ULTRA RAPID MEDICAL REFERENCE, by J. Hancock
ORGANIC CHEMISTRY MADE RIDICULOUSLY SIMPLE, by G.A. Davis
CLINICAL CARDIOLOGY MADE RIDICULOUSLY SIMPLE, by M.A. Chizner
PSYCHIATRY ROUNDS: PRACTICAL SOLUTIONS TO CLINICAL CHALLENGES, by N.A. Vaidya and M.A. Taylor.
MEDMASTER'S MEDSEARCHER, by S. Goldberg
PATHOLOGY MADE RIDICULOUSLY SIMPLE, by A. Zaher
CLINICAL PATHOPHYSIOLOGY MADE RIDICULOUSLY SIMPLE, by A. Berkowitz
ATLAS OF MICROBIOLOGY, by S. Goldberg
ATLAS OF DERMATOLOGY, by S. Goldberg and B. Galitzer
ATLAS OF HUMAN DISEASES, by S. Goldberg
ORTHOPEDICS MADE RIDICULOUSLY SIMPLE, by P. Tétreault and H. Ouellette
ATLAS OF ORTHOPEDICS, by P. Tétreault, H. Ouellette, and S. Goldberg
ANATOMY OF THE SOUL, by S. Goldberg
IMMUNOLOGY MADE RIDICULOUSLY SIMPLE, by M. Mahmoudi
CLINICAL BIOSTATISTICS MADE RIDICULOUSLY SIMPLE, by A. Weaver and S. Goldberg

Try your bookstore. For further information and ordering send for the MedMaster catalog at MedMaster, P.O. Box 640028, Miami FL 33164. Or see http://www.medmaster.net for current information. Email: mmbks@aol.com.